On my first reading, I was immediately struck by the refreshing, crisp style of this text. On deeper reflection, I was aware of the author's professional research and compassionate approach to an increasingly difficult problem within our society. Infertility is a problem, and infertile couples have few companions. Who cares about the infertile? Themselves, and their family, or course; two national self-help groups and some practitioners. But society at large? The National Health Service? Not at all! And yet, I know of no other single medical condition that afflicts such a large percentage of our population. Plato (428–348 BC) in his Dialogue *Symposium* stated that 'human nature is desirous of procreation ... for conception and generation are an immortal principle in the mortal creature.' After all, overcoming infertility is probably mankind's earliest cry for help ['Give me a child else I die' – Rachel, Genesis 39:6]. Help is not easy to find, and for some it arrives too late. Infertility management is riddled with confusion, inefficiency and contradiction. This book is a clear and precise guide through the maze. Perhaps more than any other couples, those suffering infertility need to help themselves. I firmly believe that strong motivation and a self-help attitude drives infertile couples to achieve their goals sooner and more efficiently. This book is indeed a companion for and to infertile couples and, when it is time finally to put it down, I believe its readers will do so with a sense of gratitude to its author.

SIMON FISHEL, PH.D. (CANTAB) FCPS,
READER, OBSTETRICS AND GYNAECOLOGY
DIRECTOR, *CARE*

Your Essential
INFERTILITY COMPANION

ANNA FURSE

Thorsons

Thorsons
An Imprint of HarperCollins*Publishers*
77–85 Fulham Palace Road,
Hammersmith, London W6 8JB

The Thorsons website address is: www.thorsons.com

First published by Thorsons in 1997 as *The Infertility Companion*
This updated edition published by Thorsons, 2001

10 9 8 7 6 5 4 3 2 1

A catalogue record of this book
is available from the British Library

ISBN 0 00 711954 2

Printed and bound in Great Britain by
Creative Print and Design (Wales), Ebbw Vale

For Jack, who stuck by me through thin,
and Nina who was born against all odds.

Contents

Acknowledgements

Regarding both editions of this book, I am indebted to Dr Ruth Curson at the Fertility Unit, Kings College Hospital, for her enormous help with medical information. My special thanks for additional medical advice goes to Dr Virginia Bolton, Dr Susan Waterman, Dr Wang Ling, Susan Lee Tanner ITEC MiiPTI, Olivia Woolfe Lic Ac Mbac, Carl Awty of ORGANON and Simon Fishel, director of CARE. Jennifer Hunt and Sue Emmy Jennings contributed their precious time and invaluable insights from the counsellor's perspective, whilst Tiffany Black was a fount of general knowledge and good ideas. Many other people's expertise has fed my research, and I am particularly grateful to Clare Brown of CHILD, both Juliet Tizzard and Jess Buxton of PROGRESS and Berkeley Greenwood of NIAC. Heartfelt thanks too for the generous help of Andrew Boyd, Deborah Lowe, Kay Lyn, Elspeth Morrison, Lucy Bland as well as all those people undergoing infertility treatment who have shared their experiences with me and let me use their own words.

Among the authors quoted, particular thanks to Tim Appleton, Pamela Armstrong, Jacqueline Brown, Carl Djerassi, Timberlake Wertenbaker, Benjamin Zephaniah, Lynn Segal and Jack Klaff. Of the countless people who have given advice and encouragement, thank you to the staff at the Hammersmith Hospital, Belinda Barnes, Sarah Cable, Gowan Clewes, Barbara and John Deegan, Serono Laboratories, the HFEA, Margaret Jeffery, Pippa Kennedy, Sophie Henderson, Julia Johnson, Carla Lamkin and Nicky Klaff.

Lastly I would like to thank my editor Erica Smith, a fellow traveller, for her expert advice and guidance, Marylin Virgo for assisting research for the second edition, Barbara Vesey for correcting the manuscript with such a keen eye and my publisher Wanda Whiteley for her unstinting support of the project from its first edition to this one.

Foreword

Most of us take our fertility for granted. Many of the readers of this book will have planned their lives carefully and will have decided when to have a family. Infertility is the most frustrating hitch to encounter because it removes control and forces people to be dependent on outsiders. Dreams and plans are all disrupted. People lose confidence in themselves and no longer trust their relationships or their ability to make decisions at work.

Going through infertility treatment can be demoralising. It can be physically painful and tiring. There will be times when one will feel powerless and out of control. For many it will end without having a child.

It helps to have up-to-date, accurate information about the treatments on offer, so one can ask the right questions and make decisions. Information and knowing the limits of what one is prepared to go through are the keys to regaining control.

But it is not just about facts and figures. Coping with infertility also involves coping with many difficult emotions.

It helps to hear first-hand from people who have experienced the process. As doctors, we forget that what seems logical and right to us may seem incomprehensible and frightening to others. It is a relief to know that others have trod the path and had similar experiences and difficulties.

Anna Furse offers a personal view of using infertility services. Her book is well researched, up to date and easy to read. There is a wealth of practical detail, combined with sensitive and thought-provoking insights. It truly is an Infertility Companion.

DR RUTH CURSON, M.A., M.B., B.CHIR.

Introduction

In the warm kitchen
two women are sitting
confiding failings, fears.
One woman is me.

...like an egg I'm saying
one minute tough enough
to withstand anything, next
a fingertip could crack me...

The other woman is literal –
she'll have no truck with metaphor
No *she's saying* No you are not
an egg   You are a woman

and yes, my literal friend,
I guess you are right,
but I'm a woman thinking egg
and staggering under its weight.
JACQUELINE BROWN, *THINKING EGG* (LITTLEWOOD ARC, 1993)

When I was asked to prepare this revised edition, almost 5 years on from researching the first, my publisher suggested some slight updating of certain sections. As soon as I began my fact-checking however, I realised how nothing less than an overhaul of certain sections would be necessary. Since its first publication we have a new Labour government who have pledged major reforms to Adoption law and at the time of writing are responding positively to the constant pressure of fertility awareness campaigns for fairer NHS funding. So things are showing signs of improving. In addition, alongside much needed reforms in the pipeline, reproductive technology itself is advancing daily, with better drugs, new techniques and significant scientific breakthroughs with the potential for revolutionising our future reproductive landscape – which in turn continue to feed heated ethical debates. My last word in the first edition was "the media reported that a scientist had successfully cloned a sheep". That was 1996. In 2000 the first rough draft of the Human Genome Project was completed. And with these two milestones the media continue to focus our attention more on the macabre aspect of reprogenetics present and future than any potential social, medical and psychological benefits. Within the context of collective anxiety about endorsing eugenics individuals get demonised for using science and law to help them create families. Journalists play on people's notions of the 'selfishness' of the infertile. It is vital that society debates the pros and cons of scientific advancement, and its potential abuses. However, sensationalism will never help or support the individual suffering from the lack of and yearning for a child.

Infertility[1] should rank as one of life's major traumas alongside bereavement and divorce. Unfortunately it isn't generally recognised as such. Most people have no idea of the suffering it causes, how it can take over your life, undermine your sense of security and your confidence in the future. In short, for anyone who knows the anguish of involuntary childlessness: it's crisis time. So if you're reading this it's likely you're feeling terrible. I think I know how you feel. I've been there. I'm neither a medical nor ethical expert but a layperson whose eyes have been opened by my own experience of ART (Assisted Reproduction Technology, or Technologies). My partner and I were totally unprepared at the time for our high-tech baby-making efforts. We stumbled into the fertility clinic still reeling from the shock of diagnosis. I was panicked, desperate – and very ignorant. We were both instantly launched on a steep and often bewildering learning curve.

Facts about subfertility tend to reach the patient in fragments. A word from a Consultant here, a fleeting conversation with a fellow-patient there.

Available literature on the subject is mostly written by male doctors whilst a patient's perspective is usually to be found tucked away in the pages of support group newsletters. In all my own years of trying, of tests and eventual treatment I needed – and couldn't find – a book which could help me cope with the *totality* of our experience. I wanted information *and* consolation. I wanted to know in detail what happens medically *and* emotionally. I wanted to know my options and my rights, who were my allies and where to locate them. And then I needed to make sense of why eruptions of public furore about ART could so intensify my private, voiceless hell. Once I began to locate a personal crisis of infertility in its social, economic and cultural context I also began to realise how it is that subfertile people are misunderstood, silenced and marginalised. The fact that we are distressed and crisis-driven can isolate us, crush our spirit and turn us into victims. But being victims makes us into bad patients. We shouldn't have to suffer in silence, nor should we feel that if we do speak out we have to justify our choices of action to anybody else. Rather, we need to convert our sense of powerlessness into self-determination, and convert those around us into a dependable support system. I hope this book might help.

By a river that flowed through a mountainous province of Japan, there lived a childless woodcutter and his wife. To all the children in the neighbourhood they were known with warm affection as Grandmama and Grandpapa, because, in spite of their poverty, they always remembered to keep a part of their small meal for the hungry young people who came to greet them daily. It grieved them greatly that they were childless and always as their young friends turned homewards and their gay voices showered the evening air with their 'thanks' and 'goodnights', they would slide the paper screen doors of their small house together and pause, silent and dejected, as if they could not bear to enclose the emptiness within.

THE PEACH BOY: JAPANESE TALES AND LEGENDS (EDS HELEN AND WILLIAM MCALPINE; OXFORD UNIVERSITY PRESS, 1958)

The majority of people in the world get babies through love or accident, assuming a right to breed. Subfertiles don't have the luxury of Nature on our side. We have to work extremely hard at reproduction, our eyes pinned open. Because the decisions we face are so tough and our prognosis so uncertain, many of us weigh the route of medical intervention against pressing issues such as over-population, scientific ethics and sexual politics. And there's no shortage of reasons for opting to remain childless, although on closer examination some of these might not prove as rational as they first seem. For example:

There's a terrifying crisis of thousands of unwanted babies born each year in poorer countries and adoption is a vitally important option to consider. Yes of course, and many childless couples do just this, but it's unfair to cast infertile people as human sacrifices in the cause of population control.[2]

Infertility is a way of 'naturally' reducing the population and therefore shouldn't be medically treated. Follow this argument through and you find yourself in an ethical landscape where we cease to use medicine for curing any fatal illnesses or for any prolongation of life.

ART is a male conspiracy designed to keep women trapped in their biological destiny of motherhood. Well, the field is certainly male-dominated and often traditionalist, but most women who opt for fertility treatment do so voluntarily, having searched deeply their own motives for wanting a child so badly. And children really do have the right to be born *wanted*.

Arguments against intervening in an infertile 'fate' may actually be rooted in deep anxieties. For some reason the treatment of infertility makes people feel extremely uncomfortable. We are nervous of science trying to outdo Nature and (justly) wary of the arrogance of doctors 'playing God'. We eat highly processed foods and meat bred in artificial environments (albeit with increasing scepticism). We enjoy the most sophisticated technological commodities and our thirst for the freedom and mobility they bring is apparently unquenchable. Yet when it comes to making babies, even the most sceptical and irreligious of us can turn squeamish, easily affronted or technophobic. It's what's known in the trade as 'the yuk factor'. Reproductive science has been moving at a giddying pace and we can't always get our brains around some of the latest techniques – until they concern us directly. When we undergo fertility treatment we're forced to confront many fundamental issues. Willy-nilly, we might have to let go of previously help views or assumptions of what is both 'right' and 'natural'.

Conception – and subfertility – are at the best of times Nature's lottery, yet infertile people often feel irrationally responsible for their affliction. We may blame ourselves for past decisions, lifestyles or medical negligence. We can't make a family 'naturally' so we may begin to doubt our *right* to have one. This feeling isn't helped by economic realities. We don't only face the prospect of childlessness but a system which regards our desire for a child as a 'luxury' not a necessity. You will probably have to pay for your treatment and it doesn't come cheap. So it's not just medically, but socially and financially that the odds are stacked against us.

I believe we have the right to map out our reproductive future. ART is the other end of the telescope from birth control in the sense that it means to have *control of our reproductive potential*. And we surely have the right to assert that with the help of medical science our desire for a family is a relatively simple and perhaps achievable one. This book is written with these issues in mind, knowing that what its readers really need is to find out all they can about what may lie ahead, empowered and undaunted.

As this book's subtitle suggests, being an ART-user includes familiarising yourself with a range of tests, technologies and therapies, both physical and psychological. I include chapters on complementary medicine as well as counselling because I would encourage you to think holistically about the process, taking care of both your body and mind. A healthy body keeps your energy levels up and helps to counteract depression. A positive mental attitude enables you to make decisions, keep a grip and handle the stresses of disappointment. I don't bombard you with statistics and League Tables. Why? Because these not only present misleading information but tend to get you into a kind of obsessive thinking which can dislocate you from the real questions to ask your helpers, the clinic and yourselves. So try instead to hold on to the idea that you are a human being, not a statistic. In our own case, ignorance was ironically merciful. We never knew that at my age I stood only a 3–9 per cent chance of having a 'take home baby' using my own eggs. I had thought it was 25 per cent and was never disabused of this notion by the clinic. If we'd known the 'true' prognosis we may never have proceeded with our two IVF attempts, finally producing our miracle-baby girl when I was 42.

You will find the Appendix on UK clinics is designed to help you take all kinds of practical factors into consideration when choosing where to go. Details such as carparking facilities may seem irrelevant – until you try rushing for an early morning jab before work and are frustrated by your journey and so doubly stressed by the time the hormones kick in. Again, it's about being prepared. You might not be in a position to choose the ideal situation, but at least you will know what questions to ask and how best to organise yourself – for much of fertility treatment is about time-and-life-management.

Then there's the question of networking. There are plenty of organisations and individuals passionately devoted to improving the lot of the childless. Some of these are professional subsidised charities and some are attached to religious organisations. But there's also a web of self-help activity out there: people beavering away voluntarily, generating information from their kitchen tables amidst busy lives, talking to strangers on helplines, tirelessly passing on their own experience of childlessness and its resolution to others. I hope some of the information I've collated might simplify your research and help save your precious energy for trying to make a baby.

Finally, this book is designed to be read either sequentially or as a reference manual. So you can skip any passages or chapters which aren't relevant to you. I sincerely hope it will offer some guidance, sustain you through the ups and downs and remind you of an important and easily forgotten fact: you are not alone.

Good Luck!

Anna Furse, December 2000

---

1. Please note that 'infertility' is actually rare and means a total absence of reproductive function. Much more common is a dysfunction or 'subfertility'. I use the terms 'infertility' and 'subfertility' interchangeably to denote any impairment in a man's or woman's reproductive system.
2. Interestingly enough, recent figures about birth rate trends in the UK suggest that approximately 20 per cent of women born in the 1960s, 1970s and 1980s will remain childless (twice as many as their mother's generation) and that as a result by the year 2011 the child population will be seriously outnumbered by the retired population.

CHAPTER **1**

Where Do Babies Come From?

Be realistic, plan for a miracle.

ANONYMOUS

① You and Your Reproductive Body

1. The Woman

There are three phases in a woman's reproductive life: childhood (before), maturity (during) and menopause (after). We measure these phases in eggs – their quantity, quality and availability. At birth the ovaries, incredibly, contain around 400,000 eggs. But thousands will degenerate, and only about 400 develop in maturity to become part of the monthly ripening and shedding dance that is menstruation. By the menopause, any remaining eggs are 'past their sell-by date' and the body decides to cease ovulation altogether.

So, unlike men – whose bodies continue to make sperm throughout their lives – women are born (literally) full of our reproductive potential, and our lives are governed by a biological clock. This clock starts ticking at the onset of puberty, when the traffic of reproductive hormones starts circulating from the brain to the ovaries and back again, telling the body how to anticipate fertilisation by sperm and how to deal with the consequences of this happening or not.

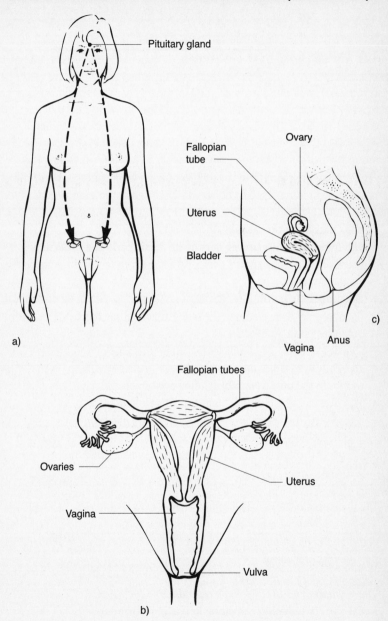

Figure 1: The female reproductive system. a) The mind and the body are one: the pituitary gland in the brain sends out hormones to the ovaries to stimulate ovulation. b) The reproductive organs, front view. c) The reproductive organs, side view.

Understanding How Ovulation Works: The Menstrual Cycle (Periods)

The word 'menstruation' comes from the Latin 'mensis', meaning 'month', because the menstrual cycle supposedly takes place over a period of a month. In fact the neat 28-day cycle is actually rare, and many women have regular but shorter or longer ones. Each monthly period involves a cycle of internal activity in which the ovary matures a *follicle* (sac containing the egg), an egg is released from the follicle, and the womb lining is shed. This whole process is governed by hormones produced in the *endocrine glands*.

The key players in the menstrual cycle are:
- **The hypothalamus (lower part of the brain) and the pituitary gland.** They are like 'central control', with an overview of the whole cycle via the production of:
- **Hormones (from the Greek meaning 'to stir')**, which are the chemical messengers flowing through the bloodstream telling the reproductive organs when to do what:
- **Ovaries** store eggs and follicles (which in turn send out hormones).
- **The Fallopian tubes** are active pathways – tubes which lead from the ovaries to the uterus (womb), guiding eggs down and sperm up.
- **The uterus** is the eventual home for a developing embryo. Its **endometrium** (lining) grows during the menstrual cycle and is shed if not needed (no fertilisation) through the cervix and into the vagina, which is your 'monthly bleed' (usually lasting three to five days).

The menstrual cycle actually has two phases, each lasting two weeks. First is the *oestrogen phase*: everything is geared towards the production of the egg; and then the *progesterone phase*: when ovulation takes place and the uterus prepares for pregnancy.

The key hormones in the female reproductive cycle are:
- **LH-RH: (Luteinising Hormone Releasing Hormone)**
  - produced by the hypothalamus in the brain, triggers the pituitary to release FSH and LH
- **FSH: (Follicle Stimulating Hormone)**
  - produced by the pituitary, this is the egg-maturing hormone

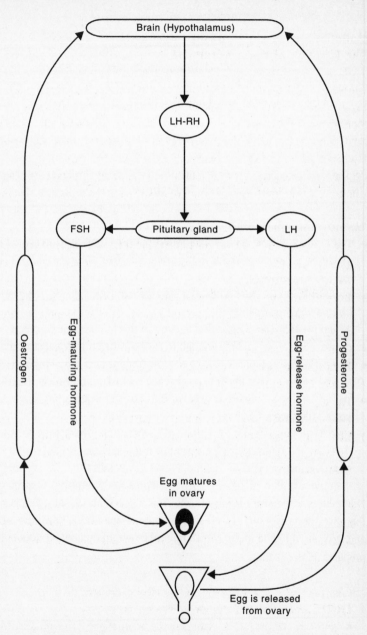

Figure 2: The female hormone axis. The female reproductive hormone system is a continuous and cyclical process. Notice the feedback process from the ovary to the brain.

- **LH: (Luteinising Hormone)**
  - produced by the pituitary, this is the egg-releasing hormone
- **Oestrogen**
  - the female hormone which triggers the reduction of FSH/production of LH, and growth of the endometrium. Produced in the ovary, it acts on the whole genital tract and breasts
- **Progesterone**
  - makes the endometrium receptive to the embryo

How the Hormones Work Together

Some months before ovulation, eggs in the ovaries mature inside follicles – little sacs containing cellular and fluid support systems for the egg cell. Each month the hypothalamus in the brain tells the pituitary gland to release follicle stimulating hormone (FSH), which acts on the ovaries to tell about 20 follicles to grow. Whilst the eggs grow in their follicles, the ovaries start producing oestrogen.

When the brain recognises that enough of this has been produced, it decreases FSH, releasing only enough to concentrate on the developmental activity of one 'prize' follicle and its egg. Oestrogen starts preparing the uterus to thicken in readiness to receive and nourish a pregnancy. The rising oestrogen levels, meanwhile, signal the pituitary to release luteinising hormone (LH), which tells the ovary to start ovulation – the release of the egg from the follicle. After ovulation, the ovaries stop producing oestrogen and switch to progesterone. This hormone is made by cells in the ruptured follicle which have been left behind. Progesterone tells the endometrium to stop growing and to become receptive to a prospective embryo. The egg, released from the ovary, leaps into the arms of the fimbria – little tentacle-like growths at the ends of the Fallopian tubes – and travels down the tube to be fertilised by the sperm, which might be swimming upwards to meet it.

A Cycle without Fertilisation

Where no sperm have arrived or managed to burrow into the egg-shell, the egg simply disintegrates and is absorbed into the body. Progesterone and oestrogen levels fall. The blood vessels in the now thick and spongy endometrium break and the womb fills with blood and broken tissue. The muscular walls of the womb contract and expel the menstrual debris through the vagina as a menstrual bleed, which lasts a few days. Then the cycle commences all over again.

A Cycle with Fertilisation

Where sperm have managed to reach the egg and one has burrowed into it, fertilisation takes place and the process of cell division immediately commences. Meanwhile, the embryo makes its way down the Fallopian tube into the uterus, where it lodges in the receptive endometrium. The process from fertilisation to implantation takes about seven days (during which time the Fallopian tube will have nourished the embryo). The moment the embryo begins to attach, it starts to produce the pregnancy hormone human chorionic gonadotrophin (hCG)). Many embryos never implant at all or are lost after implantation. This is common to both fertile and infertile women. We often never even know this is happening, since a very early pregnancy failing in this way reveals itself as a period, possibly a bit late. Why a pregnancy which doesn't implant is so distressing when undergoing fertility treatment such as IVF is that you get to know a pregnancy result weeks before you would under normal circumstances, and may have even seen your embryo(s) on an ultrasound scan.

> Day 1 of a menstrual cycle is the first day of proper bleeding (that is, red blood rather than brownish discharge). It is vital to remember this when making your own temperature charts and when trying to understand medical information, timings and general management of treatment cycles.

The following diagram shows the relationship between ovulation, fertile periods, hormone production and the condition of the endometrium.

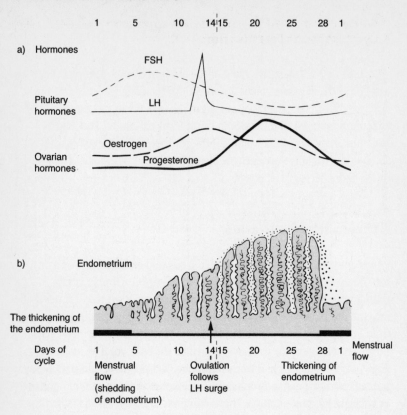

Figure 3: Hormone production, ovulation, changes in the endometrium and fertile phases of a woman's menstrual cycle. a) Changes in hormone levels. b) The shedding and thickening of the endometrium (womb lining).

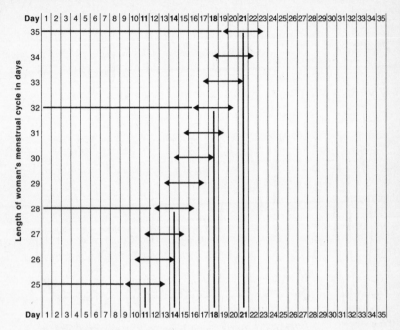

NB: Days of ovulation are in bold (Day 1 is the first day of the woman's period)

Figure 4: Fertile days in a woman's cycle. Not all women have a 28-day cycle. This chart helps to indicate when ovulation might occur in cycles of different lengths.

2. The Man

Unlike women, whose egg-producing days are limited, men start to produce sperm at puberty and continue to produce it throughout their lives at the rate of millions each day.

Many people confuse *sperm* with *semen*. But men with no sperm still have semen. This is because semen is a fluid which normally contains only about 2 per cent sperm. The rest is made up of acidic seminal fluid (produced in the *seminal vesicles*, which are next to the upper ends of the *vasa deferentia*) and alkaline fluid (from the *prostate gland* at the top of the *urethra*). These chemicals keep the sperm healthy and help to counteract vaginal acids which can destroy sperm. The vasa deferentia and seminal vesicles connect to the *ejaculatory ducts* in the prostate. These in turn empty into the urethra, which carries the sperm outside the penis on ejaculation.

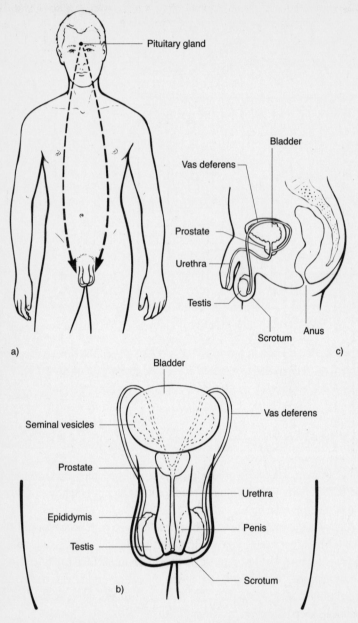

Figure 5: The male reproductive system. a) The relationship between the pituitary hormones and the testes, where sperm are produced. b) The reproductive organs, front view. c) The reproductive organs, side view.

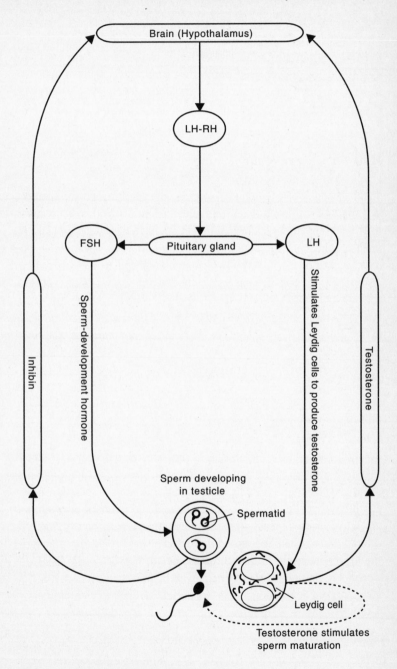

Figure 6: The male reproductive hormone axis.

The penis is an erectile organ composed of three cylinders of tissue and blood vessels. The penis hardens when it becomes engorged with blood from the veins inside these cylinders. Fertility is affected neither by the size of erection nor erection itself, but by the quantity and quality of sperm from the semen ejaculate (however, lack of erection – impotence – can of course prevent sperm from reaching the inside of the vagina).

How Sperm Are Made

The male and female reproductive organs not only complement but also echo each other. The same sex hormones are found in both systems albeit in different quantities and with different but equivalent functions. Like the woman's, the man's reproductive system is governed by hormones secreted in the endocrine glands (hypothalamus, pituitary and, in men's case, gonads or testicles). The hypothalamus starts the ball rolling by sending LH-RH to the pituitary, telling it in turn to send out FSH and LH to the testicles. Whereas in women we have seen that the hormones work on a cyclical axis, in men the hormones FSH and LH are produced simultaneously and continuously.

During the first 64 days of sperm production (*spermatogenesis*), sperm have a head and tail but can't yet swim. They are called *spermatids*. Recent research has proved that a spermatid can be capable of fertilising an egg under laboratory conditions; *see page 77*. By the time the sperm reach the epididymis (where they spend about 12 days), they mature, developing an oval head capped with an acrosome (a kind of pointed helmet with which to burrow into the egg), a body and a long tail. It swims by thrashing its tail about and pushing its head forward. Once ejaculated, the sperm undergoes another stage of development, *capacitation*. This is when the acrosome's protective 'hairnet' breaks up so that the sperm can work on cracking through the eggshell. The second the acrosome has successfully punctured the egg it releases the nuclear chromosomes (carriers of genetic codes) stored in it, causing the shell to harden itself against any other sperm invasion. DNA flows through, the two nuclei fuse and cell division starts. An embryo has begun to form.

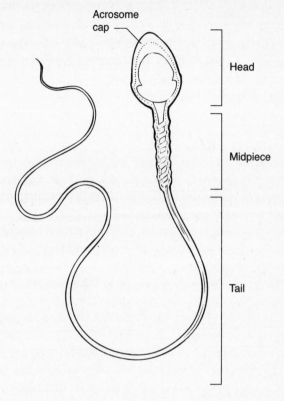

Figure 7: A single sperm. This is a fully mature, healthy sperm. Technology has now made it possible to fertilise an egg with an immature sperm.

Testosterone

Testosterone is the male hormone that stimulates the sex drive. The sex drive is Nature's way of maintaining our interest in the survival of the species, and is not to be confused with sperm or egg production per se. Testosterone is associated in the public imagination with virility, and virility (falsely) with fertility.[1] In men it makes the penis and facial hair grow and the voice break and deepen. Controlled by the hormone LH (which is the egg-releasing hormone in women), testosterone is made in the *Leydig cells*, which are tucked inside the seminiferous tubules. This process works simultaneously to the stimulus of FSH on the *Sertoli's cells*, also in the seminiferous tubules, which make sperm. Too much testosterone can inhibit the production of FSH, which will in turn reduce sperm production. So testosterone-aided body-building might make you look like a tiger and have sex like one, but it won't necessarily make you reproduce.

Sexual Intercourse

Ejaculation

Pleasure and romance aside, the male and female anatomies are superb complementary systems of near-flawless design. The human race, like many other species, is propagated by a simple action of depositing semen into the vagina. Yet before this can take place, the most intricate interplay of hormones, secretions and pulsations must take place in labyrinthine folds of tubing, tissue, organs and blood vessels, unseen and normally unfelt to us as we go about our daily lives.

An average ejaculate might deposit up to 100 million sperm into the vagina. A staggering amount when you think that all this is just for the one egg. But for millions of sperm ejaculation is only the beginning of their decathlon to reach the egg. At ejaculation begins a hazardous survival-of-the-fittest race against both time and the many obstacles which may befall them. The vagina is remarkably hostile to sperm, killing off more than 90 per cent of them with its natural acidic cleansing secretions. Of those that then make it through the cervical mucus (which they can reach in minutes) into the cervical canal, only a few hundred will survive to make it to the uterus. Many will then take a wrong turn into the Fallopian tube which isn't involved in ovulation that month. More will now fall to the wayside, so that by the time they reach the middle of the Fallopian tube where the egg might be waiting, only a few dozen survivors are left. These batter against the shell of this egg, the *zona pellucida*, until one single sperm is allowed in. There begins the process of fertilisation and cell division. This union can take place as soon as half an hour after ejaculation.

If no egg is waiting because ovulation hasn't yet occurred, for example, sperm can survive in the Fallopian tubes for about three days, where they may wait patiently until the egg appears. This is Nature's way of enhancing the opportunity for fertilisation. It actually means that you can still get pregnant if you have sexual intercourse before ovulation, and that you don't necessarily have to time it minutely.

Getting Pregnant Naturally: Timed Intercourse

When trying to get pregnant 'in bed', timing is of the essence – although doctors are divided as to the efficacy of Timed Intercourse. During preliminary stages of subfertility investigation, your GP might have asked you to keep a temperature chart to monitor your cycle and ovulation (*see page 27*). There are also DIY ovulation prediction kits on the market. They're available over the counter at chemists and can be more accurate than temperature readings since they test for the presence of ovulation hormones (LH). A prediction kit is recommended because it works in advance of, rather than retrospective to, ovulation. It is especially useful if you have irregular or infrequent periods, since it would be harder for you to establish ovulation by using a temperature chart. Another method of prediction is by observing your own cervical mucus. Mucus production tends to increase just before ovulation and the mucus to become clear and watery.

If your periods are infrequent your chances of pregnancy are reduced because you are producing fewer eggs. It is important that you take the time to establish your own cycle, as this can have an effect on both 'spontaneous' pregnancy and the medical management of any ART programme you may be put on.

The Fertile Phase of a Woman's Cycle

This is generally 14 days before the start of your period (bleeding). Eggs live one day, and sperm two to three days, so frequent intercourse just before, during and after ovulation will maximise your chance of pregnancy (*see Figure 4*).

Getting the Best Odds from Your Sperm

There are some cultural, spiritual and medical ideas about abstinence improving the quality of sperm. To an extent this is true, for sperm counts can go down with frequent ejaculation, but they do recover very quickly (within two to three days of abstinence).

Conversely, sperm quality and motility deteriorates within a few days, so too much abstinence can result in a large 'store' of useless, dead sperm.

So on balance, a couple of days without ejaculating before the woman's day of ovulation, then regular intercourse during ovulation, should offer you the best odds.

The Chances of Getting Pregnant Using Timed Intercourse

Provided you and your partner have no subfertility problems, you will stand roughly a 1 in 3 or 4 chance of becoming pregnant during each cycle.[2] Most spontaneous pregnancies will occur within two years of trying, about 80 per cent during the first year. There are ways of enhancing your chances and getting your reproductive systems into peak condition (*see pages 168–186*). However, the reasons why the majority of people conceive when they do, or not, remains largely a medical mystery and it is important not to add guilt and self-reproach to any failure to get pregnant when actively trying.

GETTING PREGNANT CHECKLIST:

Getting the egg and sperm to fertilise through intercourse requires:
Correct hormone balance for the egg to develop normally
Ovulation (the release of the egg into the Fallopian tube)
An adequate number of motile, healthy sperm
Intercourse (vaginal penetration by the penis) during ovulation
Ejaculation (male orgasm) into the vagina
Cervical mucus which is hospitable to sperm
No mechanical obstruction preventing fertilisation, for example blocked
Fallopian tubes, adhesions around the ovary

The Pressures on You of Timed Intercourse

Timed Intercourse can be a great strain on you as a couple. Sex can lose its spontaneity, women can feel desperately anxious to 'hit the moment', whilst men can feel they are having to 'perform on cue'. These factors can cause impotence, loss of libido, frustration and anger. A woman who has been taking her temperature or measuring her hormones will most probably have been counting the days – even the hours – whilst the man may well forget what time of the month it is. You wouldn't be the first couple to find yourselves having a screaming row precisely at ovulation time because of the stress involved. Chrissie Jones, in her book *The Emotional Side of Infertility*, suggests that, like animals, when trying to get pregnant we should accept separating sex-for-reproduction from sex-for-pleasure. So you can do both and not get distraught if your Timed Intercourse doesn't make the earth move.

Timed Intercourse Prescribed by Your GP

If you are under 30 years old with regular periods and having frequent sex, being prescribed a year of Timed Intercourse may be fine. If, however, you are either having infrequent periods, suspect you may be early-menopausal, or if the biological clock is ticking, you would be well advised to insist that your GP refers you for fertility investigations. Time can be of the essence. There are too many cases of women finding themselves leaving thorough investigations till too late, increasing the likely need for the more invasive treatments and curtailing their chances of getting NHS funding.

Lack of initiative on the part of your GP or advice from certain complementary practitioners to 'wait for Nature to heal you before taking a medically invasive route,' can cause serious delay to your getting started on any necessary treatment. Don't let yourself be misled by other people's agendas. Follow your own instincts. Try and impose your own deadlines for decisions or actions. Take expert medical advice, but don't lose control of your chances of ever reproducing in the process.

ⓘ Getting Diagnosed: Tests for Infertility

There was once upon a time a King and Queen, who were so sorry that they had no children, so sorry that it was beyond expression. They went to all the waters in the world, vows, pilgrimages, everything was tried and nothing came of it. At last however the Queen was with child, and was brought to bed of a daughter.

PERRAULT'S *HISTOIRES OU CONTES DU TEMPS PASSÉ* (1697; TRANS. IONA AND PETER OPIE IN *THE CLASSIC FAIRY TALES*, OXFORD UNIVERSITY PRESS)

First Hurdles

One of the first frustrations of in/subfertility can be the lengthy and complicated ways in which you will reach a conclusive diagnosis from which to survey your options. The current arrangement of the Health Service seems to conspire with the spectrum of whims, myths and prejudices amongst certain (although by no means all) GPs to mean that your fertility investigations may often only start up to 18 months later than necessary. Whilst the 'go-away-and-have-sex-for-a-year' advice from your GP might seem sensible, given the average time it takes for any fertile couple to conceive (20–25 per cent success rate in any one month) it is not such good advice to anyone who suspects they may have fertility problems because of, for example:

- past venereal disease (VD)
- Pelvic inflammatory disease (PID)
- impotence
- endometriosis
- irregular or no periods
- weight problems (anorexia or obesity)
- recurrent miscarriages
- many unprotected 'risks' taken
- age
- alcoholism
- drug abuse
- undescended testes
- torsions of the testes
- radiation treatment for cancer.

Not all of the above mean you definitely have problems, but if you are in any doubt about your ability to make a baby as a consequence of any of these factors, you should alert your GP to the urgency of your need for a conclusive diagnosis. In an ideal world, an efficient fertility assessment scenario might look like this:

8 steps in an ideal and pro-active fertility assessment

1. Active trying for a baby starts:
- Rubella Antibody Screening (at GP)
- Cease contraception
- Have regular intercourse during fertile period of cycle (ovulation identified with Basal temperature chart and/or ovulation prediction kit)
- Start taking Folic Acid (prevents Spina Bifida in babies)
- Monitor your own fitness, weight, stress, alcohol intake, diet, leisure drugs
- Quit smoking

2. No pregnancy after 6 months?:
- Visit to GP, reporting 6 months of failed attempts.
- GP starts fertility investigations:

3. Fertility tests with GP:
- Temperature charting
- Semen analysis
- Blood Test for Day 21 Progesterone levels LH, FSH within first five days of period starting

4. GP uses results to refer you: directly to an infertility specialist

5. Infertility specialist to check: Woman:
- Full endocrine (hormone) assessment
- Ovulation assessment (including scan)
- Cervical mucus test, as part of post-coital test

Man:
- Antibody assessment
- Semen analysis to include a 'swim up' test for motility

6. If both partners 'pass'[3] these: Post-coital test

7. If post-coital test 'passed'[4]: Woman to have uterine investigations:
Hysteroscopy and/or Laparoscopy (Lap and Dye) (*see pages 30–1*) to check tubal patency, condition of uterus and ovaries, presence of cysts or fibroids and/or Hysterosalpingogram (HSG)

8. Further consultation to: evaluate all results and discuss treatment options and prognosis for success

Sadly, in the UK such a straightforward procedure isn't always the case, particularly in the public sector. On the NHS many women are first referred to a Gynaecology Consultant at a local hospital. Tests are then conducted over weeks and months. Where straightforward surgery or hormone treatment is advised, this might be offered there. However, where more expensive treatments options such as IVF are advised, this gynaecologist might then refer the patient to an IVF Unit, or in some cases (as in my own) leave the patient(s) on their own, baffled consumers in the ART marketplace.

If you then find yourself in an IVF clinic, especially the better and more thorough units, you may well find some tests being repeated. Valuable time has passed. Time during which your stress and distress will have mounted. Time during which, for the older woman, you may hit or pass the NHS funding age-limit decided by your Local Health Authority.

The best thing you can do is to be pro-active. As soon as you decide to try for a baby, keep a diary of the times you have sex and, if possible, a menstrual chart and temperature chart (*see Figure 8, page 27*). This will save you and your GP time when you first tell her or him about your suspicion of subfertility. Don't stick your head in the sand. Talk about what's happening with your partner. Try to be a team, sharing knowledge and information before investigations even start. Make a health plan together, reducing or cutting down on smoking, alcohol and generally getting a sense of control over your own bodies.

It is important to remember that most of the several tests for infertility are quite routine, even the surgical ones. Some women become extremely anxious during this phase, fearing that internal investigations imply some dreaded fatal disease. Such results from investigations are rare. Far more common is to find blocked or damaged Fallopian tubes (which make up 22 per cent of all known infertility causes) or ovarian cysts, which, though alarming, don't necessarily have any bearing on your ability to conceive. The anxiety we may feel during routine infertility tests has probably to do with our deepest fears about our health in general. Added to which, a woman's reproductive apparatus is 'all on the inside', a mysterious inner landscape about which we may have felt mystified and alienated from all our lives. Our menstrual cycles may cause us pain or not, emotional turbulence or not, and we will have varying attitudes to our bleeding and what it signifies according to our culture and its menstrual taboos. What is universal is that the shedding of our womb lining after ovulation is the only tangible evidence we have of the complex and brilliant functioning of our reproductive system. For men it is different. Most of their reproductive organs are external. Their seed is visible and easily accessible. The 'seed-store' (testicles) can be seen and felt. It is this very difference which means that infertility tests for women are so much more varied and complicated than those performed on a man, and not, I repeat *not*, because the majority of infertility problems are female.

The highest single cause of infertility is male (32 per cent).

Lastly, it is important to bear in mind that, whilst each test itself is routine – that is, frequently performed – and that there is an ideal chronology to a full fertility assessment as outlined above, some tests, particularly those further down the line, will be irrelevant to your situation. Your individual histories, what is known and what is discovered along the way, will determine which tests are conducted and when.

1. Tests for Male Infertility

There are three possible causes of male infertility: hormonal, genetic or physical.

Hormonal

The human reproductive systems are controlled by a balance of hormones – chemical 'messengers' secreted by the endocrine glands (which include the pituitary, ovaries, testicles). Sometimes insufficient levels of hormones may affect sperm production. Hormone treatment may rebalance or replenish the body's natural system and restore fertility. However, not all hormone-related sperm deficiencies can be hormonally treated, in which case some of the newer IVF techniques might be advised (*see pages 60–92*).

Genetic

Klinefelter's Syndrome is an extremely rare condition where the man's chromosomes contain at least one extra X (female) chromosome, leading to low testosterone levels and usually a total absence of sperm production. The condition is currently untreatable. Where small amounts of sperm are produced, some of the newer IVF techniques such as ICSI (*see pages 76–8*) might be feasible (but the couple would have to consider the genetic implications), otherwise donor sperm would be the only option.

Physical Causes

These are basically structural problems in the tubing through which sperm flows to reach ejaculation. Causes can be previous infection, injury, hernia or prostate operations, or congenital absences of the vas deferens. Techniques exist to obtain sperm by aspiration, and usually this method would be combined with IVF.

How Are These Causes Identified?

Semen Analysis

This is the most basic test that can be carried out. The man ejaculates into a sterile container, either at home (provided you can get the sample to the hospital within an hour) or at the hospital. The sample will be measured and the following will be calculated:

a) *volume*: amount of semen ejaculated
b) *density*: number of sperm per millilitre (ml)
c) *motility*: number of sperm showing normal forward progressive movements
d) *morphology*: percentage of abnormal sperm.

A normal analysis would show the following:

a) a volume greater than 2 ml with:
b) more than 20 million sperm per ml

c) motility greater than 40 per cent (within one hour of ejaculation)
d) less than 70 per cent abnormal sperm[5]

Tests may also be carried out to check for the presence of antisperm antibodies in the semen, which may cause a 'clumping' of sperm resulting in an inability to reach the egg.

An abnormal semen test might show the following:

Aspermia/Azoospermia:	Semen containing no sperm
Oligozoospermia/oligospermia:	Semen containing less than 20 million sperm per ml
Asthenozoospermia/asthenospermia:	Less than 40 per cent of sperm are motile
Teratozoospermia/teratospermia:	More than 70 per cent abnormal in shape
Oligoasthenoteratozoospermia (OATS):	Less than 20 million sperm per ml + less than 50 per cent motility + high number abnormally-shaped
Necrospermia:	All sperm in semen are dead
Pyospermia/leucospermia:	White blood cells present, implying infection

Generally speaking, with sperm it really is the quality rather than the quantity that counts, particularly with new treatments in which a single sperm can be isolated and used to fertilise the egg (ICSI; *see pages 76–8*).

Sperm production and quality can fluctuate enormously depending on the man's health. It takes about 10 weeks for sperm to reach maturity, so an illness 10 weeks prior to testing can affect count and motility. For this reason semen analysis will always be repeated at least once if not twice over about three months, even if the first test results prove normal.

If all the above tests produce a normal result, a Sperm Invasion Test might be conducted (*see below*).

Hormone Tests

If your sperm count is low, hormone tests will be conducted via blood tests to measure:

- The pituitary hormones LH (luteinising hormone) and FSH (follicle stimulating hormone)
- testosterone
- prolactin.

Other blood tests may be done if a man is born with an absence of vas deferens to check whether he is a carrier of cystic fibrosis, since the two are linked.

Surgery

An exploratory operation may be carried out. A biopsy of the testis might be removed, to ascertain whether the testis is producing sperm. The doctors can see whether the epididymis (tube next to the testis) or the vas (leading from the epididymis to the penis) is blocked or diseased. A dye test might also be performed on the vas deferens (similar to the woman's 'Lap and Dye'; *see page 29*). This involves injecting a small amount of dye through the tube and then examining it under x-ray to see whether there is any blockage to the dye flowing through.

2. Tests on Both Partners

Post-Coital Test

At ovulation, the woman's cervical mucus becomes profuse, watery and clear. This is as a result of an increase of oestrogen produced in the ovary. It is Nature's way of creating a temporary welcome for sperm, which can normally swim through this mucus on their journey up the cervical canal to reach the egg. A Post-Coital Test checks for this.

The Post-Coital Test is conducted as near to ovulation as possible. You will have been asked to have intercourse about eight hours prior to attending the hospital. A speculum is passed into the vagina and a mucus sample taken from the cervix. The procedure is painless, but the ritual of the test itself can be a little inhibiting. After all, turning up and announcing to the receptionist that you've had your prescribed sex a few hours before is something you might understandably find embarrassing. Don't worry, they've heard it all before!

You might also find having sex by medical request very difficult, or even impossible. Try not to feel pressurised. The world won't end if you don't manage it, and you can always try again the following month. Trying to combine romance and body-fluid offerings on demand might prove mutually exclusive. Can you and your partner talk this one through and see how you can help each other get through it with the least amount of anxiety or tension – perhaps even with a laugh? In my experience, a healthy dose of 'gallows humour' throughout our infertility treatment made all the difference and helped us cope and get closer.

Post-coital testing involves examining the 'stretchability' or elasticity of the mucus and, under a microscope, the sperm population is counted and motility assessed. A normal result would show very stretchable mucus containing a significant number of active (motile) sperm, swimming in a 'forward' motion rather than on the spot.

If no sperm or only dead sperm are found in the mucus, or if the mucus itself is very thick, the test would be considered negative. A negative test is usually repeated, as several factors might have produced the result: The test might not have been timed right to coincide with ovulation, or you may not have ovulated that month. You may also have antibodies in the mucus or sperm, for which a Sperm Invasion Test would be carried out.

Sperm Invasion Test

This is to test whether sperm is able to penetrate the woman's mucus and to what extent motility is then maintained. The test is conducted at the time of a woman's ovulation. Having abstained from intercourse for 24 hours, you both attend the hospital. A mucus sample is taken from the woman's cervix and a sperm sample is produced by the man. These are placed side by side on a glass slide. Sperm activity over the next 15 minutes is then observed under a microscope.

Further checks might be carried out using donor sperm and donor mucus. This is known as a 'cross over sperm invasion test' which can help deduce antibody or other factors. If sperm doesn't even get into the mucus or stops swimming in the mucus, there may be antibodies in either or both the semen and mucus. These will be checked in blood samples as well as semen and mucus samples.

3. Tests on the Woman

Basal Body Temperature Chart (BBT chart)

This is one of the oldest 'DIY' methods of birth control as it is basically a test for patterns of ovulation. It is simple, cheap, and you can start doing it even before you go to your GP.

Ideally you should use a special fertility thermometer which shows a Centigrade scale (obtainable at most chemists). You create a chart for each monthly cycle, starting on the day your period starts (Day 1) and continuing daily until your next period begins.

Normal BBT chart

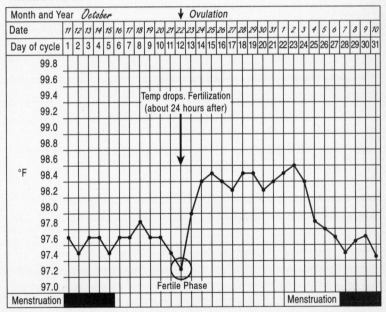

Figure 8: Basal Body Temperature (BBT) chart. A normal cycle showing a fall in body temperature at just about the time of the LH (luteinising hormone) surge, about 24 hours before ovulation, after which the secretion of progesterone will cause a slight rise in temperature (about 0.2 degrees).

The chart is made up of dates and temperature recordings. You record your temperature at the same time each morning, and fill it in the chart as a dot. You then join up the dots to show the rise and fall of your body temperature, which gives you a reading of your ovulation.

At ovulation (on the chart shown in Figure 8 between Day 12 and 14) there is a fall in temperature, swiftly followed by a rise which remains up until the next period begins. Compare the chart shown in Figure 8 with Figure 3, which shows how progesterone rises at ovulation and then falls until the next period. This is because when you don't ovulate you don't produce progesterone and your temperature will remain low. The temperature chart is quite simply noting changes in your progesterone level.

Some doctors ask that you also keep a menstrual diary either alongside or incorporated into the chart. For instance, you might wish to note the extent of bleeding, pain, mood changes, even the changes in your vaginal mucus. This information can all be useful at early stages of investigations.

Blood Tests for Progesterone

Progesterone rises a few hours before ovulation, peaks about seven days after and falls suddenly before the next period. Blood tests (sometimes taken over a few days) can detect this and indicate whether or not ovulation has occurred.

Blood Tests for Prolactin

Over-production of this hormone (which stimulates milk-production after pregnancy) can prevent ovulation. This, incidentally is why breastfeeding has been an age-old (though not foolproof) method of contraception.

Hormone Assays

These are blood tests to measure the whole balancing act of your reproductive hormones – FSH (follicle stimulating hormone), LH (luteinising hormone), oestrogen and progesterone. Prolactin and thyroxine levels might also be measured.

The 'Luteal Phase Progesterone Test' is just one of these tests. Testosterone levels in the woman will also be tested for, as it is raised in cases of Polycystic Ovarian Syndrome.

Endometrial Biopsy

Where the body doesn't produce enough progesterone after ovulation, the endometrium (womb lining) might not have developed in preparation for implantation of the embryo. Testing the endometrium is another way of checking your progesterone production.

The test is performed about two to three days before your period is due. Requiring no anaesthetic, a fine suction curette is inserted into the uterus and a small biopsy taken.

Tubal Patency Tests

There are essentially two tests currently carried out to check the condition of the Fallopian tubes.

Hysterosalpingography (HSG)

This is an x-ray of the uterus and Fallopian tubes, requiring no general anaesthetic. It can be uncomfortable, causing cramps similar to a period pain. An instrument is inserted into the cervical canal and a dye squirted into the uterus and tubes. The subsequent movement or blockage of this dye, visible on the x-ray, will indicate any obstruction, swelling, spasm or adhesions of the tubes.

HSGs are performed in the hospital x-ray department and require no overnight stay.

Laparoscopy ('Lap and Dye')

This requires general anaesthetic and hospital admission. It is essentially an operation to give the doctors a 'window' into your insides. A tiny incision is made in your navel, and the abdominal cavity filled with carbon dioxide gas, which creates space so that the doctor can get a complete picture of the abdominal cavity, uterus and Fallopian tubes.

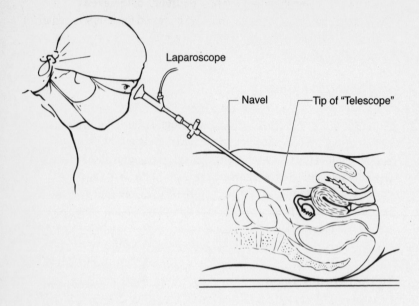

Figure 9: Laparoscopy. A small incision is made in the abdomen (at the navel) and a small telescope is inserted to allow direct visualisation of the ovary and Fallopian tubes.

A laparoscope (basically a thin telescope) is inserted into the incision and the doctor looks through it to inspect what is going on inside. The laparoscopy is a thorough test, giving a full picture of the condition of the tubes and any adhesions, the condition of the uterus including the presence of fibroids, endometriosis and the ovaries together with any cysts. During the laparoscopy, tubal patency can be tested with dye.

RISKS AND SIDE-EFFECTS OF LAPAROSCOPY

The laparoscopy is a minor operation and most women can return home the same day or the next morning. It can 'take it out of you' and you may not feel really well for a week after. Post-operative discomforts vary in degree but can include:

- pain in the abdomen
- pain in the neck and shoulders. This can be very intense. It is caused by the gas which has been blown into the abdomen. It has nowhere to escape to.

- sore throat as an after-effect of the anaesthesia
- staining from vaginal secretions which are expelling the dye used in the tubal testing
- vaginal bleeding.

Hysteroscopy

This might be carried out at the same time as the laparoscopy.

A hysteroscope is also a fine telescope, inserted through the cervix.

A hysteroscopy can be performed either under mild sedation and local anaesthetic or general anaesthetic. The hysteroscopy gives the doctor an opportunity to carry out a detailed assessment of the uterine cavity to check for any irregularities of shape (which may have caused recurrent miscarriages), fibroids, a 'septum' in the uterus (the abnormal development of a wall of tissue dividing the cavity in two) or adhesions (which sometimes form after a D and C – dilation and curettage – operation).

You should bear in mind that the above three operations can produce results which may be upsetting and which may be delivered by a doctor you don't know. Make sure you are prepared and, if possible, have your partner or a close relative/friend with you.

Ultrasound Scanning

An ultrasound scanner translates sound waves from matter into images. Fluid looks black and solid matter various shades of grey, giving strange, ghostly and pulsating images on the screen (which you may watch). Most women have at least one or two ultrasound tests during the natural course of pregnancy to check foetal development. Ultrasound is now sometimes used to check ovulation and follicle development. Abdominal ultrasound is a painless test, except for the fact that you have to drink enormous quantities of fluid beforehand and this can be very uncomfortable – and a real test of your bladder control! (The sound waves travel best through water, so a full bladder permits a view of the ovaries.) Ultrasound is usually done by passing the scanner over the abdomen. Most clinics today will favour the newer ultrasound equipment: a Vaginal Scanner. So don't be alarmed if you are asked to straddle stirrups and watch the person who is to scan you putting a condom and jelly on the scanner (which actually resembles a large penis) before inserting it.

The advantage is that you don't have to drink gallons of water and the process itself is normally quite quick and painless. If you want to be prepared as to what to expect, ask what equipment is used when your appointment is made.

(III) What Causes Infertility?

As we have seen, the male and female reproductive systems are intricate designs relying on the interplay of several factors, organic and hormonal. Many things can go wrong with them in an adult's lifetime. Some will easily be correctable with the minimum of medical intervention, some will require the help of modern medical technology, whilst some, sadly, will be chronic and incurable. Only people affected by the last factors would technically be classed as infertile. Most people actually have what is known as subfertility, meaning that part or parts of the reproductive system are impaired or dysfunctional whilst the rest of it functions normally, resulting in a reduced rather than zero chance of conceiving without medical intervention.

CAUSES OF INFERTILITY[6]

Male factor (sperm quantity/quality):	32 per cent
Hormonal:	28 per cent
Tubal:	22 per cent
Uterine abnormalities:	11 per cent
Cervical abnormalities:	3 per cent
Unknown/'unexplained':	4 per cent

Infertility Is a Random Condition

Sub/infertility can strike anyone at any time. There is often no rhyme or reason why some people are infertile and others not, and problems with fertility can feel like a cruel trick Nature has decided to play. It is important to understand the many things which can go wrong and can interfere with achieving a 'spontaneous' pregnancy:

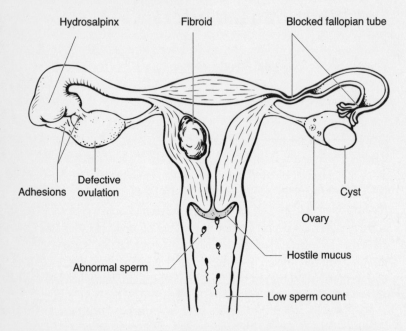

Figure 10: Causes of infertility. What can go wrong, and where.

Main Things Which Can Go Wrong

- Men may have problems in producing sperm, sperm of the right quality or quantity
- Men may have structural problems in their reproductive organs (such as absent vas deferens)
- Men may have problems with ejaculating
- Women may fail to ovulate or have difficulty in ovulating (due to polycystic ovaries, early menopause, hormonal disorder, weight problems, stress, effects of shock, etc.)

- There may be hormonal problems such as thyroid disease (affecting both men and women)
- Women may have endometriosis
- Women may have blocked Fallopian tubes or damage to other reproductive organs such as ovaries and uterus
- Women may have Polycystic Ovary Syndrome (PCOS)
- Women may have cervical mucus which is hostile to their partner's sperm
- There may be the presence of toxins, allergies and nutritional disorders affecting both partners.

Some Key Causal Factors

Tubal Damage

One of the most common causes of female factor infertility is tubal damage due to past infection. Infection may be caused by sexually transmitted diseases, or from the insertion of an IUD or from bacteria being passed from either the anus or urethra into the vagina. When infection travels up the vagina, into the uterus and on into the Fallopian tubes, the condition is known as Pelvic Inflammatory Disease. PID can be extremely painful and sometimes require hospitalisation. It is normally treated with antibiotics. Other damage to tubes may be caused by adhesions from previous surgery such as an appendectomy, and from endometriosis. Tubal infection itself often leaves the tubes permanently scarred.

Many women now in their forties with chronic tubal damage may be victims of the IUDs we inserted with gay abandon in our youth, perhaps thinking them less chemically invasive than the Pill. The truth was that the insertion of a foreign body into the uterus not only temporarily inhibited conception but frequently caused permanent sterility. When the Dalcon Shield, issued with such enthusiasm in the 1970s, was discovered to be a huge cause in PID, the device was banned in the First World. It continued to be exported to the Third World, a contraceptive which was in fact sterilising women en masse.

The spectrum of sterility in our world then has three aspects, all of them menacing. The first is the involuntary sterility that has been spread by disease throughout the developed world and throughout its colonies and dependencies, with which we have not begun to deal; whether the rich spend fortunes in trying to reverse it or the poor simply suffer it, it carries out its inexorable work. The second is the sterility we choose for ourselves in preference to continuing the struggle to regulate our own fertility. The third is the sterility we persuade others to accept because we doubt their capacity to regulate their own fertility or because we do not trust them to do it. Among the dubious achievements of the twentieth century, along with total war and the neutron bomb, will go our character as the sterilising civilisation.

GERMAINE GREER, *SEX AND DESTINY – THE POLITICS OF HUMAN FERTILITY*

(SECKER AND WARBURG, 1984)

Sexually Transmitted Diseases

These are various and increasingly widespread. A recent survey of a London infertility clinic found that 69 per cent of patients suffered from genito-urinary infections. Apart from PID, infection can also cause ectopic pregnancy and early miscarriage. In men, infection can cause a blockage of the ducts in the testes and affect sperm production. Chlamydia is a particularly problematic VD since it is far less easy to detect than, for example, gonorrhoea (where heavy discharge is produced). It is wise for both partners to have tests at an early stage of infertility investigation to check whether either or both of you might be harbouring any infections, and to get them treated instantly.

Endometriosis

Endometriosis is a relatively common chronic condition women suffer and about which the medical profession remains perplexed. The uterus largely remains a mystery and research has not yet managed to define either the cause or definitive cure.

In endometriosis, deposits of cell structures which appear to be womb lining are found outside the womb, in nearby organs, in the abdominal cavity and the tubes. Endometriosis causes internal bleeding and pelvic pain. Pain may be experienced during intercourse, periods, ovulation and other times. Endometriosis may leave scar tissue and adhesions. Diagnosed through laparoscopy (*see page 29*), endometriosis is currently treated by surgery or through the use of ovulation-suppressing hormones.

Polycystic Ovarian Syndrome (PCOS)

Approximately one in five women has polycystic ovaries, which should not be confused with PCOS. PCOS is a condition in which a woman has polycystic ovaries together with other symptoms. Polycystic ovaries contain at least 10 small cysts, some of which may contain eggs, some of which may be secreting hormones, and others of which may be dormant. In PCOS the body is in a condition of hormonal imbalance. Women may develop skin conditions such as acne and facial hair (caused by an excess of testosterone). Periods may be irregular or absent and miscarriage may occur due to higher than normal levels of LH. Overweight plays a crucial part in the condition. PCOS is more common in obese women, and some women with polycystic ovaries only develop the actual syndrome when they put on unusual amounts of weight. PCOS is normally treated with hormone drugs and advice to reduce body weight.

Causes

Clomiphene Citrate is successful in inducing ovulation in 70–85 per cent of cases, but where patients don't respond then gonadotrophins might be prescribed. If there is no positive response to drugs you may be advised to have Laparoscopic Ovarian Surgery (*see pages 29–31*) to remove some ovarian tissue. The latest advance technique is called Ovarian Diathermy. This involves laser or what is called monopolar electro-cautery and simultaneously destroys parts of the ovary and repairs it. Results are apparently extremely positive. An article in the magazine *Pathways to Pregnancy* (No 3 Summer 2000) states that studies of 35 women show that ovarian diathermy had a 90 per cent ovulation success rate with a 69 per cent conception rate. The technique does carry a certain amount of risk – irrevocable damage to the ovary leading to ovarian failure – but has the advantage of a being a one-off treatment with no risk of ovarian hyperstimulation from drugs.

Meanwhile, treatments on the market to relieve some of the more unpleasant symptoms of PCOS include Vaniqa Cream by Gillette which treats unwanted hairgrowth and Ins1 or Insmed which helps to control insulin levels.

Stress

Apparently rabbits – perhaps the fastest breeders of the animal kingdom – don't procreate easily when there is undue noise. Even when well kept and fed, many animals in captivity are far less fertile than in the wild. This suggests that an unnatural environment may cause animals stress and that this stress may in turn affect their reproductive function. We live today in extremely stressful environments, divorced from Nature. There is enormous pressure on us to reproduce, and the failure to do so despite active trying invariably results in emotional tension. Added to which, infertility investigation and treatment re-locates us from a 'natural', private reproductive environment to that of a hospital or clinic. Is there a catch-22 here? Are you infertile because you are stressed or stressed because you are infertile?

It is by now widely acknowledged that there is a relationship between psychological and physiological stress, and that hormone function is crucial in this. Reproductive hormones can be affected by CRH (corticosteroid-releasing hormone) and beta-endorphins – the hormones which are increased by anxiety, depression or stress. Beta-endorphins affect brain perception. They act as chemical messengers and appear to alter pain perception, temperature regulation, eating, learning, respiration and cardio-vascular control.

Whilst the 'hunches' of many patients and practitioners is that there is a definite correlation between stress levels and infertility (particularly in the case of 'unexplained' infertility), research has yet to prove this conclusively. The results of a recent Hammersmith Hospital study showed no significant difference between women with unexplained infertility and women with tubal problems. They only noted stress levels rising during an IVF cycle – hardly surprising – and a very slight decrease in sperm count before and during.

Smoking

Cigarette smoking in men lowers testosterone levels, affecting the development, density and motility of sperm. Women smokers are more prone to early menopause and early miscarriage, whilst studies show that smoking can affect infant birthweight and that heavy smokers have a higher risk of producing babies with brain damage and foetal malformations such as cleft-palate and hare-lip.

Alcohol

There are different schools of thought on this. Some would advocate complete tee-totalism when trying to get pregnant, whilst others say that drinking in moderation has no adverse effect on fertility or pregnancy. There is obviously a big difference between occasional social drinking and alcoholism, but it is worth noting what alcohol at worst can do.

It is proven that alcohol is a direct testicular toxin, causing atrophy of the seminiferous tubules, loss of sperm cells, and an increase in abnormal sperm. It can affect sperm concentration, output, morphology and motility. Research has established that 80 per cent of chronic alcoholic men are infertile and that it is the most common cause of male impotence (hence sometimes known as 'brewer's droop'). Alcoholism in women has been proven to affect their babies. There are common characteristics associated with children born from what is known as Foetal Alcohol Syndrome (FAS). These include: poor growth both in the womb and post-partum, congenital malformations such as unusual facial features, cleft palate, cardiac defects, abnormalities in the nervous system and mental disability.

Weight Problems

Being underweight can cause infertility, as can sudden weight loss. This is for several reasons. Firstly, hormonal. Your appetite control centre is situated in the hypothalamus, the same part of the brain which is so significant in stimulating the reproductive hormones which get the ovaries and testes to do their job. Its function as an appetite-regulator may well interact with its reproductive function. It is very common that anorexic women often stop menstruating altogether.

Women with Polycystic Ovarian Syndrome tend to put on weight as a result of the condition as well as this weight factor contributing to their hormone imbalance. Control of obesity in such cases sometimes improves ovulation.

Ultrasound scanning, egg collection and embryo transfer can be extremely difficult to perform on a severely overweight woman since it becomes harder to locate the ovaries accurately. For one's own safety and to maximise your chances it is therefore wise to regulate your weight.

Diet

Poor diet, food additives, malabsorption of nutrients in the gut, vitamin and mineral imbalances and high levels of toxic metals in the body can have serious consequences on your fertility (*see page 180*).

Environmental Hazards

Research now suggests that certain heavy metals such as lead, mercury, cadmium, aluminium, copper and selenium can have adverse effects on fertility. Chemicals such as Organochlorine (OC) and pesticides (including DDT, lindane, dieldrin and aldrin) are particularly harmful. Latest evidence suggests that OC pesticides have oestrogenic properties. The BMA published research in 1992, reporting the dramatic decline in sperm density and quality in industrialised countries (by 50 per cent) in recent years, attributed to oestrogens in the foodchain derived from chemical pesticides and possibly the water supply being polluted with oestrogen from contraceptive pills excreted in human waste matter. The main culprit, DDT, has been banned in the West for many years, but is still widely used in developing countries, whilst OC pesticides may well be in the foods we import.

Research in this area has also revealed that certain occupational hazards related to chemicals in the work environment make certain categories of men at risk of low sperm counts (such as working with insulation materials in lofts, working with some paint products).

Heat

Overheating the testicles by wearing restrictive clothing can have a dramatic effect on sperm production and motility. Nature has situated the testicles outside the body to keep them cool, and has created a natural thermostat by enabling the testicles to retract into the body for warmth in conditions of extreme cold. Research has suggested that dispatch riders, for example, are a male group who have a significantly reduced sperm count due to a combination of lead fumes and the tendency to sit for long hours in tight leather clothing which may overheat the testicles.

Unexplained Infertility

The fact that this condition is called 'unexplained' says it all. It may hit people at any time, whether or not they already have children. In mainstream medicine it remains a mystery, whilst alternative practitioners may treat it as both a product of imbalances of energy or of malnutrition, severe vitamin and mineral imbalance, allergy or the presence of harmful toxins (*see pages 183–4*). The term 'Unexplained Infertility' may therefore be referring to what medicine can't yet conclusively diagnose rather than to some sinister and chronic 'barrenness' in the woman.

Dr Ruth Curson at the Fertility Clinic at King's College Hospital in London says that 10 per cent of women coming to the clinic with 'unexplained' infertility problems show higher than normal FSH levels, again suggesting a relationship between hormone levels and infertility.

Infertility and the Older Woman

Whilst men are technically fertile as long as they are producing sperm, it is a fact of life that women are fertile from menstruation onwards and then infertile following the menopause. Whilst egg production may continue right through to the menopause and this may not start till their mid- to late forties or early fifties, these eggs may be of poorer quality with less chances of fertilising properly. The blunt facts are:

At the age of 35 a woman is half as fertile as a woman of 21
At 40 she will have a 1 in 3 chance of being infertile
At 41 a 2 in 3 chance

The HFEA Annual Report (1996) includes a statistic table looking at the relationship between a woman's age and the live birth rate. It shows that, whereas the live birth rate for women using their own eggs decreases rapidly from the age of 35, with a steep decline after the age of 39, the live birth rate for older women using donor eggs (which must come from women under the age of 35) is equal to that of a 25- to 29-year-old. This data confirms the 'sell-by-date' theory that older women (who may still be producing eggs and superovulate abundantly) produce poorer quality eggs.

Risks of birth defects also increase dramatically with age. However, many women prove the statistics wrong (this author included!) and can be helped with both complementary approaches and ART.

Early Menopause

Some women's ovaries run out of eggs long before their middle age; this is known as an early menopause. Whilst common, the cause or causes haven't yet been determined. Experts suggest that such women may have been born with a severely depleted supply of eggs or that they develop a condition in childhood which may destroy many eggs at puberty. There is some speculation that early menopause may be caused by antibodies to the ovary. Sometimes the cause may be genetic, such as in Turner's Syndrome where a baby girl has only one of the normal pair of X chromosomes. Turner's Syndrome can result in very few or no eggs and, occasionally, no ovaries. Since the body's oestrogen production would be consequently low, HRT is prescribed to put the brakes on the premature ageing effects of menopause.

(IV) Your Options

Once you have reached a diagnosis, your Consultant will present you with a picture of the options available to you. Sometimes there may be a choice of alternatives and you will need to discuss these fully so that you really understand what each treatment means. Sometimes a treatment might not be available locally and you will need to decide whether you can cope with travelling to the nearest treatment centre. Sometimes you may decide to try one option to begin with and then switch to another if it doesn't work for you. Remember to keep a sense of control over what's going on. Don't feel you are being persuaded into a certain course of action because the clinic you first attended happens to offer just one suitable treatment and not another (which may be more suitable). You may go through a period of questioning and dilemma, but it is certainly better to take time to make decisions you feel happy with than to rush headlong into something which may be costly physically, emotionally and financially, only to regret it afterwards. Finally, mainstream medicine may not be the answer for you at all, or you may want to find out if complementary therapies might work for you in combination with hormone treatment or surgery. You may want to read Chapter 5 of this book before committing yourself to anything.

Common Sub/Infertility Treatment Options

Male Factor: (that is,
low sperm count)

Hormone treatment
Surgery
Assisted Conception using own
sperm (IVF, ICSI or IUI)
Use of Donor Sperm in DI or IVF

Female Factor:
difficulty in ovulating

Ovarian stimulation with hormone
drugs

blocked tubes

Surgery
IVF

not producing own eggs
womb problem or no womb

Egg Donation
Surrogacy (with own eggs or
surrogate's)

genetic problem

Donor eggs or sperm (IVF, IUI)
Genetic Screening

You may of course decide that, rather than undergo any treatment, you
would prefer to pursue adoption (*see Chapter 6*).

1. Testosterone is actually present in small doses in women.
2. *NB:* Comparable, in fact, to the average success rate of one IVF cycle.
3. That is, tests reveal no hormonal or structural problem
4. That is, tests reveal no hormonal or structural problem
5. World Health Organization criteria
6. Data from 'Infertility' Postgraduate Update Series 1995 Edition (Reed Healthcare
   Communications Publication).

CHAPTER ②

State of the ART

*The day I saw the title of Van Steirteghem's grant proposal, 'ICSI vs SUZI'
I was intrigued. It sounded like a lawsuit, or maybe a wrestling match.
It was the first application REPCON had ever received from Belgium.
By the time I'd put down the last page, I was certain of our Board's approval.*

*I'm not a fan of acronyms, but ICSI and SUZI appealed to me – cute
children's names. Especially SUZI, until I learned that it stood for* sub-
zonal insemination, *a procedure for inserting sperm just below the zona
pellucida, and then abandoning it to its own devices. In the end I favoured
ICSI. It wasn't because of its formal definition,* intracytoplasmic sperm
injection, *the direct injection of sperm into the egg's cytoplasm.
For successful fertilisation, the spermatozoon has to get inside the
cytoplasm of the oocyte. If you're going to do it, I thought, you might as
well go* all the way. *What convinced me more than any other practical
considerations was that ICSI offered the much more alluring mnemonic:*
I can still inseminate.'

CARL DJERASSI, *MENACHEM'S SAME* (ZURICH: HAFFMANS VERLAG, 1996)

① Assisted Reproduction Technologies: Treatments Explained

Ex ovo omnia [everything from an egg]
WILLIAM HARVEY, *DE GENERATIONE ANIMALIUM*, 1651 (QUOTED BY DR SIMON FISHEL IN THE CATALOGUE TO THE 'ANGELS AND MECHANICS' EXHIBITION 1996)

You've Come a Long Way, Baby

Infertility is probably as old as human history. Certainly the human mind has always been obsessed with the idea of fertility. From prehistoric Goddess worship to the cult of the Virgin Mary (donor inseminated by God?), from tribal puberty rites to Maypole dances, people have aspired to encourage the reproduction of the species by creating optimum psychological, spiritual and medical conditions within their communities.

Like so many technological innovations, advances in Assisted Reproduction have moved with a giddying pace in the 20th century. But the scientific mind was curious enough about where babies came from to discover the Fallopian tubes as far back as the 3rd century BC! Meanwhile myths surrounding human development persisted. In the popular imagination the human being was pre-formed and contained in miniature in either the egg or the sperm. It wasn't until the 18th century that *epigenesis* – the idea of the progressive development of the individual from a formless mass – was first seriously introduced following observation of the development of a chick egg.

Some key moments in the history of fertility treatment since the 19th century include:

19th century:	Karl Dernst von Bayer, published in 1822 *The Developmental History of Animals*, proving epigenesis
	Cell theory propounded
	Discovery of oestrogen
20th century:	First 'ventroscopy' (precursor to laparoscopy) by Ott (1901) involving blowing air into peritoneal cavity to allow surgeons to visualise the internal organs
	'Genes' first coined by Danish biologist (1909) Wilhem Johannsen
(1920s–1950s):	Pituitary gonadotrophins and ovarian steroid isolated
	Progesterone isolated from corporea lutea
	Testosterone isolated from testes
	Ovulation proven to occur mid-way between menstrual periods
	'Gynaecological coelioscopy' (laparoscopy) perfected
	First human ovule extracted by coelioscopy
	Molecular structure of DNA discovered
	First claim to fertilised eggs *in vitro*
	First attempts at cooling embryos (cryopreservation)
	Recognition that tubal infertility may be 'treated' in rabbits
	Recognition that tubal infertility may be 'treated' by IVF
1960s:	Advances in ovulatory drugs
	Endocrinology of fertility/infertility began to be refined
	Birth control pill
	Early stages of human fertilisation first described
1978:	Birth of first human after IVF (Louise Brown)
1980:	First human birth after IVF using drugs for ovarian stimulation
1984:	First birth after cryopreservation
	First birth using egg donation
1986:	First pregnancy after removal of sperm from male reproductive tract
1990:	First birth using microinjection technology (SUZI)
	First pregnancies from successful biopsied human pre-implantation
1992:	First birth with intracytoplasmic sperm injection (ICSI)
1995:	First births with a spermatid (unformed sperm)

It is worth noting that since 1985 the IVF success rate has almost doubled, from a live birth rate of 8.6 per cent per treatment cycle to 14.1 per cent per treatment cycle in 1994.

> If the Birth Control Pill gave us sex without reproduction, ART has given us reproduction without sex.

A Perspective on Treatment

Technically speaking, apart from successful tubal surgery, infertility is not actually *cured* but *treated*. Chemical and surgical intervention merely create the appropriate conditions for a pregnancy to occur. But good old Mother Nature, still mystifying even the most advanced scientific minds, has the casting vote. I believe it's important to hang on to that idea, because when all is said and done, your doctors will be using Science to work *with* Nature during the course of your treatment. If you lose respect for Nature and awareness of the mystery and miracle of it all, you are in danger of allowing your whole psyche and body to become over-medicalised. That's not to say that a good dose of pragmatism isn't essential to help you decide on, monitor and manage your own treatment. A balanced and informed perspective on the entire process can only help you remain in control. But the consequences of getting obsessed with the mechanics, not least statistics, can be to over-endow the medical profession with the power to give you a baby and cause immense anger and frustration if it doesn't. The fertility wizards aren't Gods but experts with a specialist knowledge and some extraordinary technology to play with on your behalf.

You should bear in mind how relatively new the whole field is. A treatment being confidently offered by a fertility specialist is part of a long and continuous process of enquiry and experiment. Whilst many treatments are proven to work with absolutely no harm to mother or child, you are entering a new and rapidly expanding area of medical research. You may or may not have strong feelings about being a part of this continuum. The important thing is that you don't allow yourself to be swept up by the profession's enthusiasm for the available technology and make sure you fully understand your prognosis and the specific treatment or treatments offered to you.

Assisted Reproduction is controlled in the UK by Government legislation (the Human Fertilisation and Embryology Act of 1990) and monitored by the Human Fertilisation and Embryology Authority (the HFEA). However, this doesn't mean that a uniform method of treatment exists. Like any field, ART encompasses many styles and approaches. So, for example, whilst there is a medical consensus on the basic procedure of In Vitro Fertilisation (IVF), clinics may differ widely in their administration of drugs, blood-test monitoring and frequency of scans. Furthermore, not all clinics offer all the available treatments (indeed, the opposite is the case: *see pages 245–75*), so it is wise to make sure that the best treatment for you is being offered by the clinic to which you have been referred, not simply the best they are licensed to offer. You may have a case for moving clinics. Make sure you are satisfied with both the diagnosis you have been given and the treatment being advised.

Finally, Assisted Reproduction is a profession with its own mavericks, its stars and its quiet diligents. The director of each clinic and the doctors and consultants they employ will influence both treatment style and its environment. These people and their team will become a vital part of your treatment experience. At worst they might make you feel like a cog in their machine, another minion in their empire or a statistic for their records. This is clearly not good for you. At best, however, you will feel respected as an individual, your varying emotional needs will be understood and you will begin to feel as though you and the medical team become collaborators in helping you get pregnant.

There is this whole incredible team of wonderful people all beavering away at trying to get you pregnant. It's really important to hold on to who is actually making the baby, and who the parents are or will be. Not the Consultant, not the Embryologist, but you and your partner.
WOMAN UNDERGOING IVF

Sub- and Infertility Treatment Options[1]

1. Tubal Surgery
2. Andrological Surgery
3. Ovulation Induction
4. Hormonal Treatment to Improve Sperm Production
5. Insemination (with husband or donor sperm)
6. GIFT (own or donor eggs and sperm mixed outside body and immediately returned to Fallopian tube)
7. In Vitro Fertilisation (IVF) (with own or donor egg or sperm – mixed outside the body, fertilised *in vitro* and returned to the womb) and together with:

   Sub-zonal Insemination (SUZI) – single sperm injected inside the zona or 'shell' of the egg

   Intracytoplasmic Sperm Injection (ICSI) – single sperm injected into the cytoplasm of the egg

   (MESA) Epididymal Sperm Aspiration – sperm removed directly from the epididymis using microsurgery – or PESA – sperm retrieved using a needle

   Testicular Sperm Aspiration (TESE) – sperm removed directly from testis

   Spermatid[2] – unformed sperm removed from the testis and injected into egg

   Zygote Intrafallopian Transfer (ZIFT) – embryos transferred into Fallopian tubes

   Assisted Hatching (shaving outer shell of egg)

   Pre-implantation Genetic Diagnosis (embryo screening for genetic disease prior to embryo replacement)

   Cryopreservation (embryo freezing)

   Embryo Transfer (ET) – fresh or frozen embryos from own or donor gametes

   Surrogacy ('straight' – husband's sperm and host's eggs; or 'host' – with couple's embryo(s) produced using IVF)

   Donor Placenta (currently being researched)

1. Tubal Surgery (Laparotomy)

Approximately 20 per cent of female infertility problems are due to damaged Fallopian tubes. Fallopian tubes are extremely small and delicate (picture thin spaghetti) with a sensitive lining containing little hairs (called cilia) which create currents through which the minuscule egg can be met by the even smaller sperm. Fallopian tubes also nourish the fertilised egg on its journey down into the uterus. Previous infection (from, for example, miscarriage, abortion, venereal disease, appendicitis, difficult delivery of a baby) can cause adhesions, scarring and sometimes total blockage. Fluid may also be present – a condition known as hydrosalpinx. When tubes haven't been damaged by infection, deterioration may simply be the result of normal wear and tear in older women.

Tubal microsurgery involves opening up the inside of the tube and/or removing any permanently damaged portions. It is rarely recommended in cases of extreme damage, and whilst it can succeed in unblocking either or both tubes, the proper functioning of their internal lining may be beyond repair. However, tubal surgery can be successful in cases of only light adhesions (imagine clingfilm) or sterilisation reversal. Surgery may be advised when you have:

- Adhesions around the tube (due to endometriosis or inflammation)
- Blockage or scarring at outer end of the tube near the ovary
- Blockage where the tube meets the uterus.

  also where:

- You have endometriosis possibly affecting the tubes
- You seek the reversal of sterilisation.

Tubal surgery shouldn't be taken lightly. It is a major abdominal operation requiring at least one week's hospitalisation and six weeks convalescence. In certain cases it will be performed via a laparoscopy, which avoids large incisions in the abdominal wall and consequently reduces the stay in hospital to a matter of days. Whilst statistically a relatively safe form of gynaecological surgery, it isn't always recommended over and above IVF because of:

- the risk of an ectopic pregnancy
- the pain and discomfort during convalescence following the operation
- the higher overall rate of success of IVF.

However, where tubal damage is minimal surgery can be the only long-term 'cure' to subfertility (sometimes resulting in fertility being permanently restored). It has the advantage of enabling a spontaneous and non-hormonally manipulated conception to occur, and is arguably less stressful than IVF.

Tubal surgery is not controlled by the HFEA and is available elsewhere than in Licensed Fertility clinics.

Standardised Selective Salpingography (SSS)

This innovative treatment requires no surgery. The procedure involves using a hysterosalpingogram (a diagnostic x-ray of the uterus; *see page 4*) in combination with catheterisation. The catheter is passed through the cervix and up into the tube opening. The tubes are then injected full of dye at high pressure via the catheter, clearing out any debris as a result. No anaesthetic is required and the procedure takes only 30 minutes.

2. Andrological Surgery (Treatment for Male Infertility)

Many of the recent advances in ART offer new hope to infertile or subfertile men. Given that sperm can now be removed from different parts of the male reproductive system, many structural problems and even impotence can be bypassed. Also, latest techniques such as ICSI mean that even poor quantity and quality of sperm needn't necessarily prevent fertilisation. Since such advances will doubtlessly overtake the older methods very soon, I will be brief. There remain certain cases where older methods of surgery or hormone treatment might still be prescribed. The most common problems and treatments include:

Structural problems treated surgically

Injury, infection, or past surgery such as vasectomies or hernia repairs can cause obstruction of the ducts through which sperm travels in the process of ejaculation. The duct carrying the sperm from the epididymis to the urethra is called the vas deferens (*see page 9*) and a man can be born with an absence of all or part of it. The operation to remove blocked parts or clear them is called an epididymovasostomy, but it has a very limited success rate.

The most success is achieved using microsurgery and where the blockage is caused by a vasectomy.

Varicocoeles (varicose veins) which can cluster round the testicle are thought to impede proper sperm function; operations to remove them can be performed.

3. Ovulation Induction (Hormone Treatment)

About 28 per cent of fertility disorders are hormonal, and at least 20 per cent of women attending a fertility clinic will have an ovulation problem. Ovulatory problems are treated with hormones, with the intention of 're-balancing' the complex interaction of pituitary and ovarian hormones (*see pages 4–8*). Hormone treatment is the simplest, cheapest and most effective form of Assisted Conception. Hormone therapy has an extremely high success rate.

I think that there's actually surprisingly little that we know about any of the things that we're doing. We've found a system that works. For instance if you give somebody Clomid and they come back a month later pregnant – which they do – I'm just overawed every time it happens! It just seems so amazing that it happens.
DR RUTH CURSON, KING'S COLLEGE HOSPITAL, LONDON

Your ovulation problem will fall into one of five categories:
1. Hormone levels are normal but the feedback mechanism of oestrogen from the ovary to the brain (normally telling the brain to decrease FSH and concentrate on developing the single follicle which will eventually release the egg) is inhibited. Usually periods have stopped or are erratic.
2. The pituitary fails to produce LH and FSH, with the knock-on effect of no oestrogen from the ovaries. Periods will usually have stopped as a result.
3. Polycystic Ovaries. With Polycystic Ovary Syndrome (PCOS) ovaries each contain at least 10 small cysts. The pituitary gland releases abnormal amounts of LH and FSH and the testosterone level is usually higher than normal. This may result in periods stopping or being erratic.
4. Hyperprolactinaemia: Prolactin (the milk-producing hormone) may be abnormally high, whilst FSH and oestrogen are lowered. You may notice

a milky discharge from your nipples and your periods will stop or be erratic.

5. FSH levels are too high and oestrogen levels too low. If the FSH level is very high, then the problem is (premature) menopause and no treatment is possible.

Fertility drugs such as Clomid can be prescribed by a GP, and in fact this is often encouraged. Most GPs, if wise, wouldn't prescribe ovulation-stimulating drugs without the advice of a clinic.

4. Hormone Treatment to Improve Sperm Production

Most male infertility can be traced to a problem of sperm production in the testes. In some cases, low levels of pituitary sex hormones can be restored by hormone treatment (for example, hCG, FSH, hMG and testosterone). A male hormone, mesterolone, is often prescribed for low sperm counts. Sometimes these drugs will be prescribed a few months prior to Assisted Conception with AI or IVF.

5. Insemination

Artificial insemination (AI) can be done either with the husband's/partner's sperm or by donor, and is one of the oldest methods of Assisted Conception. The method will only be used when there is proven patency of the Fallopian tubes. Donor sperm used by hospitals is quarantined, frozen and undergoes rigorous testing before use. If the husband's sperm is used it may or may not be with unprepared semen. Techniques for preparing sperm have advanced and with IUI (Intra-Uterine Insemination), a more closely monitored technique than simple AIH, it is washed and treated to remove debris and dead sperm before use.

AIH (Artificial insemination using husband or partner's sperm)
This method can be used when the man has a poor sperm count or low motility rate, because this method of introducing the sperm directly into the cervical canal 'bypasses' the vagina (where acidity can harm them). It can also be used when a man has a normal sperm count but is unable to ejaculate into the vagina as a result of premature ejaculation,

impotence or anatomical abnormalities. The man produces a semen sample into a sterile container. The 'neat' (untreated) sperm is then drawn up into a syringe connected to a short plastic tube. The tube is inserted high into the vagina and sperm are squirted around the cervix and inside the cervical canal. The procedure is painless and requires no surgery.

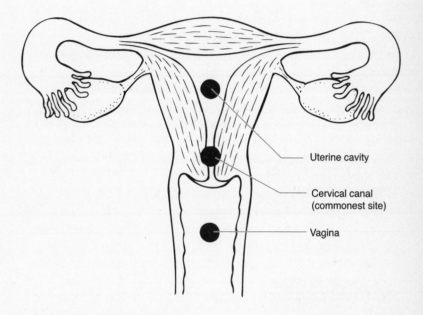

Figure 11: Sites for insemination.

IUI (Intra-Uterine Insemination)

IUI is a method which combines hormone treatment for the woman and a painless insemination procedure with the aim of assisting natural fertilisation in the womb.

IUI would not be recommended for women with Fallopian tube blockage, nor in cases where sperm count and quality are poor. It is appropriate when there is poor motility or where cervical mucus is hostile.

IUI treatment starts with egg stimulation using fertility drugs with the aim of producing perhaps two to three eggs. The follicles are monitored by ultrasound scanning; when they reach the right size, ovulation is triggered with a hormone injection. Fresh sperm is then treated by an elaborate washing process and 'swim-up' in a culture medium. The sperm which burrow into this medium will be the strongest swimmers (most motile) and it is these sperm that will be used to inseminate the woman.

Thirty-six hours after the 'trigger' injection, the treated sperm can safely be placed directly into the uterine cavity via a soft tube inserted through the cervix. The success rate is as high as that of normal fertility (that is, about 25–30 per cent).

Donor Insemination (DI, sometimes called AID)

Donor insemination involves the use of sperm from an anonymous donor. It is usually used when there is no sperm in the man's ejaculate (Azoospermia) or when there is an extremely low sperm count (Oligospermia). It may be advised when the man suffers from a hereditary disease for which he is a known carrier. It can also be used when the woman has suffered several miscarriages from Rhesus disease, in which case a Rhesus negative donor may be considered. Rarely, certain clinics may offer it to single women and lesbian couples (*see pages 238–9*)[3].

Donor insemination is widely used and is licensed by the HFEA. Because of the potential ethical, religious and emotional problems associated with it, the first stage in treatment would normally be counselling. This is essential, since there are many legal implications to the use of anonymous donor sperm, most crucially in the area of confidentiality and anonymity and the question of the child's right to know his or her origins. No DI treatment can be carried out without the written consent of both partners, and the husband or partner must consent in writing to become the legal father of any child born as the result of treatment. Once you have reached the stage of consent to DI, your treatment can begin.

DI is carried out at ovulation, which can be monitored using a temperature chart or an ovulation kit. If your cycle is regular and ovulation predictable, drugs will be unnecessary. Some clinics may determine precise times of ovulation by ultrasound. However, where periods are erratic, the fertility drug clomiphene may be used.

The medical procedure itself is painless. Insemination will either be cervical or intrauterine, as already described. Most pregnancies using DI would occur within the first six cycles of treatment. Where there is no success or where there is an additional subfertility problem in the woman (for example, endometriosis), then DI in combination with IVF may be preferred.

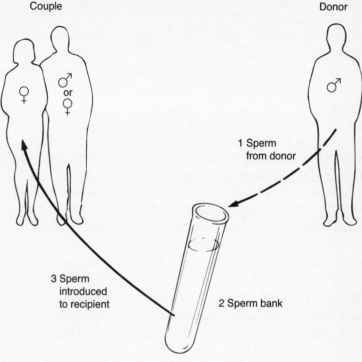

1. Sperm from donor
2. Storage, quarantine and preparation
3. AI or IVI

Figure 12: Donor insemination.

DONOR SPERM

Donors are rigorously screened before their sperm is accepted by what are known as 'sperm banks'. These banks may be either independent or attached to a hospital. Donors are also counselled about their legal position and the fact that their sperm will be undergoing much testing, and that they will have to have various blood tests, including for HIV. If they agree to the process, sperm samples are taken and measured for quality and quantity and to make sure that no infection can be cultured in the seminal fluid. Blood tests are taken to check for HIV, Hepatitis B, Cytomegalovirus and Syphilis. Swabs are taken for Chlamydia and Gonorrhoea. The donor's blood group is noted. Sperm is then 'quarantined' – frozen for six months.

The donor's blood is then re-tested, normally three months and six months later. Sperm will only be used if all three HIV tests prove negative.

DONOR MATCHING
If recipients choose, donors are matched to the male partner for race, height, skin, hair and eye colouring, blood group and general body-build.

YOUR CHOICE RE THE DONOR'S BACKGROUND
There was a time when many donors came from the medical profession itself, but now any man can volunteer to become a donor. Most people are primarily concerned about the intelligence of the donor. Also, there is continuous debate about the role religious origins do and should play in the case of both sperm and egg donation. After all, religion isn't an inherited characteristic but a culturally educated aspect of a person. However, patients' views are respected and in theory you can choose that a donor comes from a specific religious faith. In practice this can slow down the process enormously, as it may not be possible to find a suitable donor. Men from certain ethnic groups are reluctant to come forward as donors, and various infertility organisations and clinics sometimes conduct successful PR campaigns to educate the public about the need for donors. You may also be prevented from using a close relative or friend as a donor because of the emotional implications. If those assessing you regard this option as unacceptable you will have two options: First, to try and sort the situation out for yourself (that is, independent of the medical profession) or, secondly, to go through an 'ethical' procedure to try and ensure that no one will suffer if a close friend is a donor.

DONOR ANONYMITY
Anonymous donors remain so by law. The HFEA requires certain non-identifying facts about the donor to be registered (such as hair colour, build, nationality, etc.). The donor may wish to add to this list his hobbies/interests and his occupation. At 18 years of age, the child has the legal right to access this information from the HFEA (*see pages 202–3*).

DOES THE DONOR HAVE ANY RIGHTS OVER A CHILD BORN FROM HIS SPERM?
The donor has neither the right to know the child(ren), bequeath anything to the child(ren) in his will, nor any financial responsibility towards the child.

6. GIFT (Gamete Intra-Fallopian Transfer)

This technique has been developed out of IVF research into the accessing and treatment of egg and sperm. With GIFT, sperm and eggs are transferred into the Fallopian tube before fertilisation takes place. In principle this is to give Nature a nudge by introducing the eggs and sperm to each other artificially and cutting down the distance sperm have to travel through the woman's reproductive canal. It is used in cases of unexplained infertility and (less appropriately) male infertility. It can only work for women with patent (undamaged) tubes.

The procedure for GIFT is identical to IVF up until egg retrieval. That is, the ovaries will be stimulated hormonally and an hCG (Human Chorionic Gonadotrophin) injection carefully timed at the peak point of follicle development, whilst the man's sperm will have been selected from a 'swim-up'. About 36 hours after the hCG, egg collection takes place, usually by laparoscopy and under general anaesthetic. The eggs are immediately mixed with the prepared sperm and put straight back into the Fallopian tube with a very fine catheter during the same operation. GIFT can also be performed under sedation, not by laparoscopy but via the vagina and cervix. With GIFT, fertilisation occurs in its natural environment in the woman's body. Consequently, the implantation rate tends to be higher than with IVF. However, when GIFT doesn't result in pregnancy it is impossible to detect whether fertilisation was achieved or not, or to monitor embryo development if it was. For this reason IVF may be a better option since it optimises opportunities for observing whether and how fertilisation happens and to assess what might be the problem if not. Although bypassing the need for a laboratory in which to cultivate embryos, GIFT is none the less as expensive for hospitals as IVF. Given that treatment is as invasive as IVF, despite it seeming more 'natural' a process, many clinics licensed to perform both would opt for IVF. However, if you have religious or other objections to the creation, handling and discarding of embryos outside the woman's body, you may prefer it.

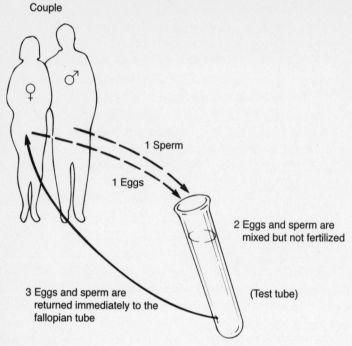

Couple

1 Sperm

1 Eggs

2 Eggs and sperm are
mixed but not fertilized

3 Eggs and sperm are
returned immediately to the
fallopian tube

(Test tube)

Figure 13: GIFT.

7. In Vitro Fertilisation (IVF) or 'Test-tube' Pregnancy

In vitro literally means 'in glass', referring to the technique of fertilising the
egg outside the body and transferring the fertilised egg (embryo) back into
the woman's womb. Louise Brown, the first 'test-tube' baby, was born in the
UK in 1978, the result of the combined efforts of Drs Steptoe and Edwards.
Since then, the technique has advanced at breakneck speed and research
associated with IVF has produced a whole array of techniques to assist
fertilisation both in and outside the body, some of which remain
controversial. IVF can be conducted using both partner's gametes, with
egg or sperm donation and, occasionally, with donor embryos. It is also
sometimes used in cases of surrogacy, where both partners' gametes are
used and the surrogate woman 'hosts' the embryo.

IVF is employed especially when there is tubal damage, but may also
be used in cases of endometriosis, where there is a poor sperm count
(Oligozoospermia), mucus hostility (mucus destroying sperm before they
get a chance to swim into the uterus), and in cases of what is known as

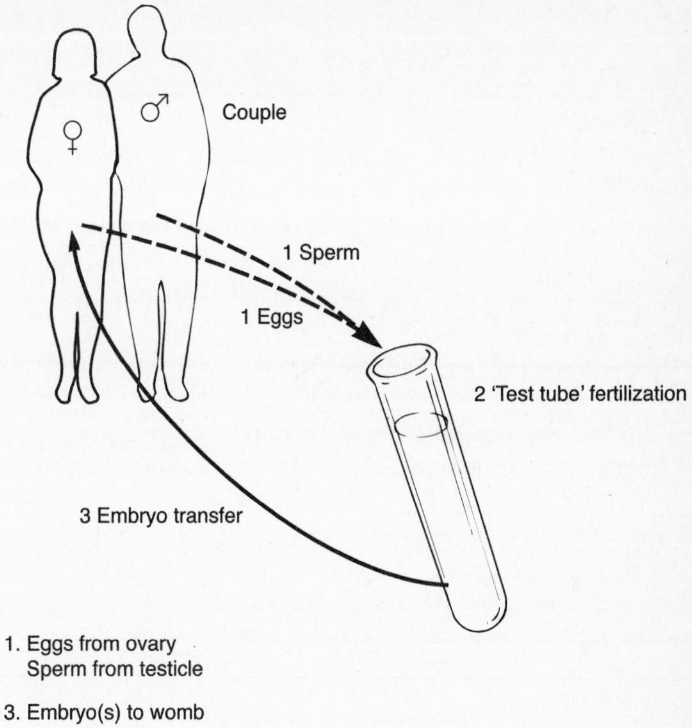

Figure 14: IVF.

'unexplained' fertility. IVF may also be used by older women experiencing a natural deterioration of egg quality and production. Where women have a premature menopause, surgery or chemotherapy, IVF may be used with donated eggs.

IVF would not normally be advised for women with severe uterine abnormalities, or for those who have had tuberculosis of the womb. Until very recently it wouldn't be advised to a couple where the man suffered poor sperm counts, but with the latest breakthroughs in sperm microinjection (ICSI, see below) specialists hope to improve the outlook for couples with this infertility factor. IVF cannot work for women who have had a hysterectomy or who cannot produce eggs or follicles. Women over the age of 42 are generally considered 'untreatable', and statistics certainly make evident the rapid decline in success rates at this age. However, there are many cases (the author's included) where IVF has worked well at this age, eggs have been plentiful and there have been a high ratio of eggs fertilising. The issue of age has continued to obsess the public imagination. The media reporting of a Doctor Antinori in Italy who managed to get a 63-year-old woman pregnant with IVF (using donor eggs) caused a furore, and both doctors and the public continue to debate the ethics of treating post-menopausal women. If you are over 40 your first hurdle will be getting accepted for treatment, and your second (at which you will invariably fail) getting NHS funding for this treatment. For a guide to the cut-off policies of various clinics, see the Appendix ('A User's Guide to UK Clinics', page 245).

IVF involves five key stages of treatment for the woman:

1. Suppressing the action of your pituitary with hormone treatment.
2. Stimulating egg production with hormone treatment.
3. 'Collecting' your eggs with surgery.
4. Fertilising the eggs 'in vitro'.
5. Replacing the fertilised egg or eggs (embryos) in your womb.

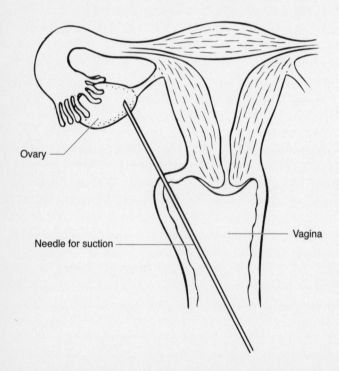

Figure 15: Egg collection or retrieval. This is usually done via the vagina by passing a fine needle through the vaginal wall and gently aspirating the eggs back down it.

The man's contribution is to provide sperm both during the testing stages and on the day of egg collection.

Following initial consultation and acceptance by the clinic for IVF, a series of tests will be conducted. Depending on how thoroughly you were tested for infertility prior to referral for IVF, these may include a hormone profile, Rubella antibody screening and perhaps a laparoscopy for the woman. In addition, some clinics may carry out a hysteroscopy (HSG) to examine the uterine cavity. The ovaries may also be scanned by ultrasound for positioning and accessibility. For the man there will be a full semen analysis, sperm-wash and 'swim-up' test. Some but not all clinics would also conduct Hepatitis B and HIV screening for both partners.

On acceptance for IVF you should be fully informed about the technique being used and your chances of success. You should (although this isn't always the case) be offered counselling at this stage. You will be asked to sign forms stating your consent to the use of your eggs and sperm (or of agreed donor gametes) to treatment, to the use of your embryos or gametes in research, and to storage. Your consent to disclose details about your treatment to your GP or anyone else who needs to know may be asked. You have the right to refuse the use of your embryos or gametes for research, but many people are happy to contribute to the advances of ART in this way.

IVF treatment normally begins either at the start of a (menstrual) cycle or in the fourth week of the preceding cycle, the precise dates of which you would have agreed with the clinic. An entire treatment cycle from commencement to pregnancy test normally takes between six weeks and two months. You will need to be very committed to treatment during this time, which will include periods of intensive daily injections, timed ultrasound scans and precision-timed surgery. Many first-timers are unaware of the kind of commitment involved and try to juggle too many things at once during treatment, only adding to their stress. So be prepared and be realistic about what treatment will require of you. You can negotiate start dates for each attempt with your clinic, and certain phases of the treatment such as the 'suppression' stage ('sniffing' or injections) you can extend by choice if, for example, you want to take a holiday prior to the intensive phase of treatment.

A typical IVF cycle would be divided into 7 Stages.
The time frame starts from the first day of a woman's period, culminating in embryo transfer approximately 3–4 weeks later. By the 5th to 6th week of an IVF cycle you should have the first pregnancy test. If this is successful, then you will be closely monitored during the next few weeks of your pregnancy.

STAGE 1: Down Regulation
Drugs are given to suppress the pituitary system, rendering the ovaries inactive. The man would also be giving sperm samples for 'swim-up' and other tests.

STAGE 2: Ovarian stimulation
Following an ultrasound and bloodtest to check that your ovaries have been suppressed, you would be given hormone treatment to stimulate egg-production via superovulation injections.

STAGE 3: Monitoring of egg development
From about 6 days after you have started your superovulation injections,your hormone levels will be closely monitored to check your oestrogen levels and vaginal ultrasound scans will be performed to assess the development of follicles on the ovary.

When scans show the follicles are the optimum size, you will prepare for egg-collection. You will be given a different hormone injection of hCG which triggers the final maturation of the eggs which would normally lead to ovulation. This injection is often called the 'midnight injection' as it is carefully timed for between 34 and 36 hours before eggs are to be collected.

STAGE 4: Egg and sperm collection
You and your partner will attend the IVF clinic. He will give a sperm sample, having been asked to abstain from sexual intercourse for two days prior to this. You will either have general or local anaesthetic and your eggs will be retrieved using a hollow needle attached to an ultrasound probe. If you are conscious you will be able to watch on a screen. Sometimes eggs might be collected by laparoscopy or by needle aspiration. The actual operation is short, and normally after a short rest you will be able to return home and carry on as normal. You may experience strong soreness in your ovaries and abdomen. You will probably (but not always) have been given antibiotics to ensure against the risk of infection.

You should be told how many eggs were collected before going home.
NB *Not all eggs will fertilise so this is at this stage no indication of how many embryos might result.*

STAGE 5: Fertilisation

Collected eggs are immediately put into a culture medium (which includes your own serum taken from previous bloodtests) and incubated for between 4 and 24 hours before being mixed with fresh (sometimes frozen) semen which has been prepared, washed and counted. The culture is now incubated. Fertilisation normally takes place within the next 24 hours. Your embryos will be carefully observed at 18 hours by which time the first signs of fertilisation can usually be detected. At approximately 48 hours, cell division will have started and two or more cells be present, occasionally more. Depending on what the embryologist observes, and whether embryos appear healthy and normal, you would probably be contacted by the IVF clinic and asked to come for:

STAGE 6: Embryo Transfer

You will be briefed by the doctor on how many eggs fertilised, how many appear usable and you will be consulted on how many embryos you wish to have put back. The maximum allowed by UK law is 3. There are pros and cons which the doctor should discuss clearly with you about how many embryos to go for. Whether or not there is a history of multiple births in your families will play a part in reaching a decision, and you must be aware that whilst two or three embryos increase your chances of pregnancy, they also increase your chances of multiple births.

Embryos are transferred without anaesthetic through the cervix into the uterus, using a catheter. This moment is one of the real perks in an otherwise stressful procedure.

> You are wide-awake and will be shown your embryos on a monitor screen. It is nothing short of awesome. It is one of the great privileges of ART that you are offered visual access to your potential child(ren) a mere 48 hours after conception. However, this imaging of the unborn can also make it very hard to bear if treatment fails. For these little microscopic structures, while by law not yet 'life' may have become deeply etched in your psyches.

Following embryo transfer you will probably be asked to lie down for a short time and then be allowed home and advised to carry on a normal routine. You will be given progesterone and further injections of hCG to help the embryo implant in the uterus.

Some women feel absolutely fine at this point and go straight back to work. Others may instinctively feel it unwise to overdo it and prefer to lie down. Follow your instinct here as there are no hard and fast rules. The important thing is to do the right thing for you as you are about to enter the hardest phase of IVF treatment: waiting for a pregnancy result.

STAGE 7: <u>Pregnancy result</u>

If you haven't started bleeding you will go to the IVF clinic for a blood or urine pregnancy test. You should be given the result that day. If the blood test detects the pregnancy hormone Beta hCG then you are pregnant and will be asked to come back in a couple of weeks for an ultrasound scan and possibly a further one a couple of weeks after that. If your pregnancy continues normally you will be advised on antenatal care. If you are not pregnant and haven't had any bleeding, you will be warned that bleeding is going to occur within days.

An Unsuccessful Cycle

If you are amongst the majority of women who are not pregnant after IVF*, then you should be given a proper consultation at which you should expect a thorough assessment of the failed IVF cycle by the Consultant and a prognosis on further attempts and possible variants in your next treatment. This is an important time to be pro-active, rather than to let yourself be so overwhelmed by your sense of failure and disappointment that you let decisions be taken for you. Your opinion, your questions, even your suggestions should be part of this evaluation. Normally you will be asked to wait for another two menstrual cycles before your next attempt. In certain cases you may be allowed to try sooner. The reason for the time in between treatments is to give your ovaries a rest, since they will have taken quite a bashing from superovulation drugs. You may feel very depressed and may need counselling (*see pages 130–6*).

---

*   Given the average 25% success rate per cycle

Things Which Can Go Wrong and Interrupt Treatment

- You may not respond to the suppressing drug.
- You may not produce any follicles.
- You may produce follicles but no eggs.
- Your eggs may not fertilise.
- Sperm on the day of egg collection may be much poorer than in previous sperm analyses.
- Your embryos may fail to develop normally.
- Your ovaries may become 'hyperstimulated' by the hormone treatment.

If any of the above happens during your treatment it will be discontinued and, depending on your prognosis, you will be advised when you can resume treatment. When paying privately, most clinics offer a financial refund for interrupted cycles. Interrupted cycles are extremely distressing but not necessarily an indication that you are chronically incapable of getting pregnant through IVF. Be sure that you fully understand what went wrong and, if possible, why. Remember, particularly if things go wrong on your first attempt, each problem that arises will give your Consultant and doctors a more complete picture of you as an individual and guide them in how to adapt treatment at the next attempt.

Things Which Can Go Wrong Even After a Pregnancy Result

- Your embryos might implant but you miscarry within weeks.
- Your pregnancy may occur in your Fallopian tube (ectopic pregnancy), which can be very dangerous and which may need to be removed surgically.

A 'Low Positive' Pregnancy Result

The pregnancy hormone measured in your blood is interpreted either as a number, for example 50–0, or as a word 'positive' or 'negative'. A result which falls between 0 and 50 or between negative and positive is called 'low positive'. It means that your pregnancy hormones haven't properly kicked in, which could be due to several factors – late implantation, attempted but failed implantation or ectopic pregnancy. A 'low positive' result means you have a 50/50 chance of pregnancy and will probably know within days the result, either through the onset of a period or with scans and blood tests.

Side-effects in IVF Treatment

It is axiomatic that the male-dominated profession of infertility specialists will want to underplay the side-effects of all the hormones women pump through their bodies during the course of IVF. It is also probably true that in your ardent pursuit of a baby, you yourself will tend to underplay any harmful or painful effects. You will not only have invested a lot of yourself in the treatment (emotionally/financially) but may also be frightened of anyone preventing you from continuing treatment. This is neither healthy nor sensible. It is prudent to look at the possible side-effects full in the face and ask yourself whether or not you are prepared to take your body through what can be both physically painful and emotionally turbulent.

What to Expect to Feel During IVF Treatment

The following checklist is a rough guide only. Not everyone will feel all or even any of the following symptoms:

At 'suppressing' stage (cf menopause), for example:

- hot flushes
- sweating
- mood swings
- vaginal dryness
- giddiness
- headaches
- night sweats
- feeling 'high'
- depression
- insomnia

at superovulation stage (cf PMT):

- tearful
- anxious
- irritable
- volatile
- hot
- stressed
- bloated
- painful or mildly sore ovaries
- 'flu'-like symptoms
- bouncy

at hCG

- elation
- trepidation

after egg collection

- drowsy
- sore ovaries
- bloated abdomen

after embryo transfer/progesterone

- mood swings
- bloated abdomen
- sore breasts
- sore ovaries

Risks

This is a matter of some controversy. Infertility specialists will all vouch for the fact that there is little risk in IVF apart from the rare cases of ovarian hyperstimulation (OHSS), estimated at 1–5 per cent of all patients. However, it is worth noting that one cycle of IVF may stimulate the ovaries to produce an amount of eggs equivalent to 1–2 years of natural ovulation! Some experts suggest IVF may be responsible for early menopause, since so many eggs from an ultimately finite supply are 'unnaturally' released per treatment cycle.

OVARIAN HYPERSTIMULATION (OHSS)

Superovulation drugs can sometimes overwork and cause the ovaries to become temporarily swollen from their normal size (about that of an apricot) to anything up to the size of a football. OHSS is a serious condition. There is a build-up of fluid in the abdomen, thorax and even the sac surrounding the heart. In extreme cases the shift in body fluids can result in a thickening of the blood. There can be thrombosis in the veins or arteries leading to possible heart attack, stroke or loss of limb. Whilst extremely rare, it can be fatal. To be forewarned is to be forearmed. So be aware of the symptoms, as not all out-patients staff will know how to diagnose the condition:

I went to my local doctor and hospital when I started to feel unwell. Nobody had seen the condition before! I had to tell them to do a scan to see what my ovaries were like. I was then told my diagnosis was probably correct. Thank goodness I'd read everything in sight about infertility!
ROSEMARY HILL (TV PRODUCER)

Symptoms of OHSS

- painful, bloated and sore lower abdomen
- nausea and vomiting
- shortness of breath
- weakness and feeling faint
- reduced urination

  NB: If you feel any of these symptoms you must contact the hospital immediately.

ECTOPIC PREGNANCY

This is a serious condition which can affect a pregnancy whether or not you have had fertility treatment. Ectopic pregnancies occur for reasons not yet fully understood. An ectopic pregnancy means a pregnancy where the embryo has implanted outside the uterus in sites where it cannot grow or be nourished. In 96 per cent of cases this mis-located implantation will be the Fallopian tube, but embryos have been known to grow in the ovary, (occasionally) the abdominal cavity outside the womb or in the womb but very near where the tube joins it. An ectopic pregnancy is ultimately unviable as the embryo cannot develop outside of the uterus or where there isn't room for it to grow (as in the case of implanting high up in the womb too near the Fallopian tube). An ectopic pregnancy can give a positive or negative pregnancy result depending on whether the embryo has survived or perished at the point of hormone testing for pregnancy.

Ectopic pregnancies can be life-threatening since they cause internal bleeding if they continue to grow. If an ectopic pregnancy has been identified, immediate surgery is necessary. Formerly this involved removal of the Fallopian tube, but recent techniques include abdominal surgery to remove the ectopic alone, leaving the tube behind. Other methods involve removing the ectopic by laparoscopy, or injecting the ectopic under ultrasound guidance with a drug called methotrexate to terminate it.

What Causes Ectopic Pregnancy?

Women prone to ectopic pregnancy are usually those with tubal damage or endometriosis. Scar tissue, torsions and blockage in the tubes can prevent the fertilised egg from completing its journey into the uterine cavity. Ironically, however, ectopic pregnancies can occur as a result of IVF treatment. An embryo transferred into the uterus can (for reasons still being researched) leave the uterus and settle elsewhere. This is why a good IVF clinic will carefully monitor your pregnancy in the first couple of weeks.

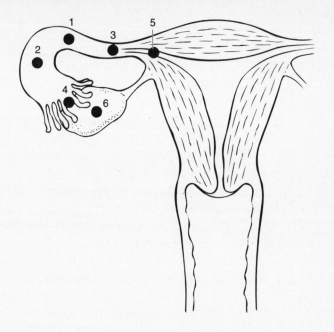

Figure 16: Most common sites for ectopic pregnancy.

Since an ectopic surviving outside the uterine cavity might continue to
show a pregnancy in blood tests (and you continue to 'feel' pregnant), a
scan would be the only way of detecting a very early ectopic. Ectopics can be
detected very early (within two to three weeks of egg collection) by repeated
blood-testing for the pregnancy hormone hCG.

Symptoms of Ectopic Pregnancy
Abdominal pain, pelvic cramps, spotting or bleeding.

CANCER
In 1995 the newsletter *What Doctors Don't Tell You* published an article
on cancer risks in infertility drugs based on research conducted in the US.
It reported that in 1993 the US Food and Drug Administration (the FDA)
required fertility drug manufacturers to add ovarian cancer to the possible
adverse reactions indicated on their products such as Clomiphene (Clomid)
and menotrophins. This was following the results of 12 American studies on
the risk factors of ovarian cancer, which found that women who had taken
fertility drugs were three times more at risk than fertile women. There are

two main theories about ovarian cancer and its possible causes. The first is that each time a woman ovulates the surface of her ovaries is slightly damaged (thus this risk is greatly exaggerated by superovulation), and the second that high levels of pituitary gonadotrophins (as stimulated by Clomiphene) can be a causal factor.

As more and more women receive treatment for infertility, we may therefore see an increasing number of cases of ovarian cancer over the ensuing decades.
DEANNE PEARSON, *WHAT DOCTORS DON'T TELL YOU* VOL. 6, NO. 7, OCTOBER 1995

but then:

In Britain in over thirty years of using these drugs, there has never been any evidence that fertility drugs increase the risk of any form of cancer.
PROFESSOR ROBERT WINSTON, *A GUIDEBOOK FOR THE IVF UNITS AT THE HAMMERSMITH HOSPITALS NHS TRUST AND THE ROYAL MASONIC HOSPITAL*, 1995

Professor Robert Winston isn't alone in responding to this cancer scare by stating that the cancer tests conducted in the US were unreliable since infertile women *not* taking drugs are already in a higher risk category for ovarian cancer than fertile women. Furthermore, he argues, childlessness is known to increase risk of breast cancer in women, and therefore successful infertility treatment may actually reduce the risk of cancer overall. Dr Simon Fishel of NURTURE in Nottingham agrees with Winston's points whilst maintaining an attitude of caution: Fishel published a paper in 1989 entitled 'Follicular stimulation in high-tech pregnancies: are we playing it safe?'.[11] Today he stands by his assertion that the profession must continue to 'observe and research' risk factors.

OTHER LONG-TERM PHYSICAL EFFECTS OF SUPEROVULATION?
Your ovaries undoubtedly take a battering from superovulation and may feel sore and bruised, especially after egg collection. You should remain confident about one thing: however strong the hormone treatment, the immediate symptoms only last as long as you are taking the drugs. Remarkably, following a failed IVF treatment cycle your menstrual cycle should resume absolutely normal function following the bleeding at the end of the treatment cycle (although it may take a few cycles).

MULTIPLE BIRTHS

Having twins may be everything you could wish for – a double miracle after years of waiting – and many couples are overjoyed to discover a multiple pregnancy and proceed to have a healthy, happy pregnancy and trouble-free delivery. But there are risks and it is important to face them when contemplating ART.

Multiple births are a real possibility following IVF or ovulation induction. The UK multiple birth rate increased from 1 in 99.5 maternities in 1982 to 1 in 78.5 in 1993, which is a significant increase 'probably largely due to the widespread use of infertility treatments'.[III] The HFEA reported that of all IVF pregnancies in 1994, the multiple birth rate was 31.7 per cent.[IV] Whilst the *Guardian* reported on 17th November 2000 that 'about half the triplets born in the UK are the result of IVF treatment with three embryos'.

When IVF fertility treatment first began there were no controls on how many embryos could be transferred to the woman's uterus, and multiple births upwards of two were not uncommon. In the UK today the Human Fertilisation & Embryology Act of 1990 forbids that more than three embryos be transferred, and HFEA data suggests that an increasing number of clinics are choosing to transfer just two, particularly in younger women. It is of course always possible that even if only two embryos are put back, triplets may result since one embryo can split in two, creating identical twins (as opposed to twins born of separate embryos, who are known as 'fraternal'). Meanwhile, ovulation-inducing drugs alone, without IVF, can also produce multiples, whilst debate continues as to whether fertility drugs should come under tighter control. Currently GPs are being encouraged to prescribe these drugs, since they are overall a cheaper and faster way of treating a woman with a hormonal imbalance than putting her through the clinic system.

Multiple birth babies are far more likely to be born pre-term than singletons and the mortality rate is higher. The miscarriage rate for triplets is significantly higher than for singletons. The HFEA report that from their 1994 data this was 20.8 per cent as compared to 14.6 per cent respectively. Twins increase the risk of pregnancy complications, and with triplets hospitalisation from six months is likely, most certainly leading to premature birth by Caesarean. Babies will often be born below normal birthweight and sometimes with mental or physical disabilities. It is not uncommon for foetuses in multiple births to abort spontaneously, which can be distressing as well as alarming since this 'natural' selection process may involve weeks of bleeding and a possible threat of miscarriage to any remaining foetuses.

In certain cases where a multiple pregnancy is considered dangerous to the mother (for example an older woman) or one baby is showing signs of abnormality, one or more foetuses can be medically destroyed *in utero* (Foetal Selection or Termination). This involves injecting the foetal heart or the fluid in the foetal sac with toxic fluid and can only be performed after eight weeks, by which time the process may be extremely traumatising for the mother. It also carries risks to the pregnancy as a whole. Finally, it is a technique which carries with it a whole raft of ethical questions.

In short, the risks of multiple pregnancies are both to the mother and babies' health, not to mention the stress, financial and otherwise, on families with twins, triplets or more. You will need advice, support and special baby equipment. Your clinic will be able to advise you or help you to get in touch with the relevant organisations specialising in supporting people with multiple pregnancies and births (*also see Useful Addresses, page 276*).

IVF TREATMENT AT A GLANCE

1. Acceptance for treatment following tests and assessment
2. Counselling (should start)
3. Hormone treatment
   a) to suppress the pituitary
   b) to stimulate superovulation
4. Assessment of egg development (blood tests and scans)? – not all clinics do this
5. Hormone treatment:
   c) to trigger ovulation
6. Egg collection (retrieval)/sperm collection
7. Embryo culture (fertilisation)? – all eggs may not fertilise, perhaps none at all
8. Embryo transfer
9. Pregnancy test:
   If successful   If unsuccessful
10. Scans   10. Full evaluation of treatment cycle by Consultant
    Antenatal care Next attempt planned? – not all couples will want/be advised to do this

---

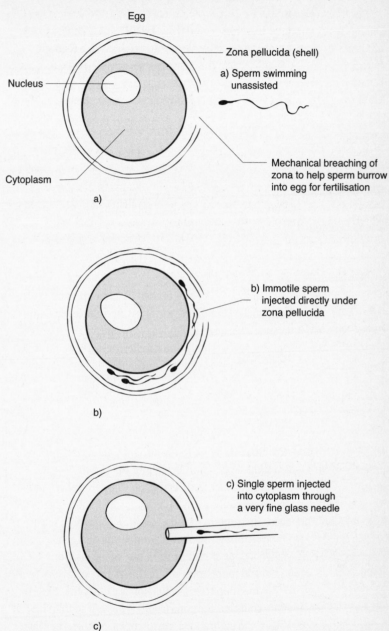

Figure 17: Three different techniques of getting sperm to fertilise an egg: a) Assisted Hatching: Partial Zona Dissection (PZD)[4] b) Sub-Zonal Insemination (SUZI). c) Intra-Cytoplasmic Sperm Injection (ICSI).

Transport IVF

Some clinics offer this service to people who don't live near an IVF clinic. It basically means that egg retrieval can be done at a local hospital. The eggs are then transported in an incubator to the HFEA-licensed IVF clinic, where the male partner gives a sperm sample, the eggs and sperm are fertilised and the embryo transfer then takes place. Whilst more convenient to certain people, live birth rates tend be reduced with Transport IVF as opposed to routine IVF.

Micromanipulation

This term refers to any IVF technique which involves bypassing the zona pellucida (shell) of the egg and includes: SUZI, MIST and ICSI. IVF may be used in conjunction with these techniques.

SUZI/MIST (Sub-Zonal Insemination or Micro-insemination sperm transfer)

This is one of several techniques used where there is a low sperm count. Egg production is hormonally stimulated and eggs are collected as with IVF. Sperm are then individually selected under a microscope and about 5–10 are picked out using an extremely fine needle; these are injected beneath the zona (egg-shell). Fertilisation is continued and embryos are then transferred into the womb as in IVF treatment. This remarkable treatment has recently been overtaken by the even more remarkable ICSI.

ICSI (Intra-Cytoplasmic Sperm Injection)

This is the treatment which is forecast to revolutionise treatment for male infertility. With ICSI, a single sperm is injected into the egg itself under microscopic control and, following fertilisation, up to three embryos are transferred back into the uterus as with IVF. What is remarkable about ICSI is that it can work even when sperm motility is extremely poor or even where there is zero motility but viable (live) sperm. It can also be used with couples who have shown a poor or non-existent rate of fertilisation following IVF attempt(s) and for couples where the sperm has to be surgically obtained. Treatment up to egg collection is exactly the same as with IVF. When eggs are collected the zona (shell) is pierced so that the cell of the egg is accessible to the eye under a microscope, and then the single sperm is injected directly into the cytoplasm.

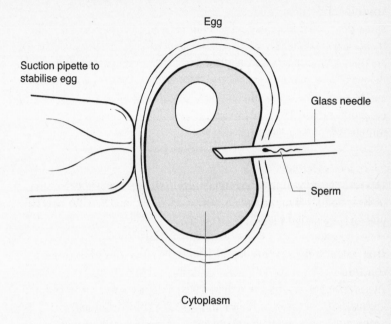

Figure 18: ICSI. This is the technique that has revolutionised treatment for male infertility. A single sperm can be injected into the cytoplasm of the egg by means of a microscopically fine needle.

ARE THERE ANY RISKS TO THE HEALTH OF THE BABY ASSOCIATED WITH ICSI?
By February 1996, only 1,000 babies had been born in Europe using ICSI, with no evidence of any increase in abnormalities. However, the piercing of the egg may lead to damage (detected during the procedure) and consequent loss of viable eggs during treatment. Some experts believe that the technique can disrupt the genetic material of the egg and also that there is a greater risk of injecting an abnormal sperm, both of which might lead to genetic defects in the baby. ICSI is legal, but as yet only a few clinics are licensed to perform it (*see 'A User's Guide', page 245*). Clinics are advising patients to be aware that ICSI remains an experimental technique; some experts suggest that regular child development assessments are advisable.

In March 2000 the journal *Human Reproduction* reported the results of a Swedish study of 1000 babies born as a result of ICSI: 'The Swedish study found that the technique did not increase the risk of congenital conditions, with the exception of hypospadias, a condition affecting the penis ... Dr Wennenholm (the leader of the study) remained positive about the technique'.

PROGRESS IN REPRODUCTION VOL. 4, 2000

MESA (Micro-Epididymal Sperm Aspiration) and Testicular Sperm Extraction (TESE)

MESA is a technique which allows sperm to be collected from men who have no sperm in their ejaculate (Azoospermia) because they have a blocked vas deferens. This is the tube which joins the epididymis (which stores sperm) and the urethra (the tubing of the penis; *see page 10*).

At the same time as the woman undergoes egg collection, the man will have his sperm removed from the epididymis either by surgery or needles aspiration. ICSI is then performed using the prepared sperm and eggs. The rest of the procedure is the same as IVF. In TESE the sperm are collected from the testis in the same way.

Spermatids

A variation on the above techniques involves using immature sperm (spermatids) removed directly from the testis and injected into the egg. Only one baby has been born in the UK (in 1995) using this method, and there followed an HFEA moratorium on any further practice.

ZIFT (Zygote Intra-Fallopian Transfer)

A zygote is another word for a very young embryo, and this technique refers to a process similar to that of GIFT, except that here it is fertilised embryos rather than gametes which are transferred into the Fallopian tubes under general anaesthetic (or by means of a catheter passed through the cervix, which can be performed with local anaesthetic). The procedure combines IVF and GIFT. Eggs are hormonally stimulated exactly the same way as with IVF and retrieved by ultrasound guidance. They are then mixed with prepared sperm and fertilised before cell division has started. They are transferred into the Fallopian tube one day later, sooner than with IVF, the theory being that the human body is still a superior environment than the laboratory in which to grow embryos and that the closer one can keep to the natural process the better. However, again, in clinics which practise both IVF and ZIFT, IVF may be recommended as it provides more opportunity to screen out embryos which are showing signs of poor development before transferring them into the woman's body. Also, it avoids the woman having to undergo two invasive and painful procedures in quick succession – egg collection and then a laparoscopy the next day.

Assisted Hatching (Partial Zona Dissection/Zona Drilling)

This is a technique designed to help the eggshell (zona pellucida) 'crack' where it has hardened during laboratory culture. The technique involves creating a gap in the zona pellucida by 'drilling' holes into the outer shell with an acid solution (Zona Drilling) or by mechanically breaking it (Partial Zona Dissection) with the aim of assisting the embryos to 'hatch'. It is thought that shell-hardening may be more prevalent in older women.

Assisted hatching would be used as an added input to IVF (although Partial Zona Dissection no longer has a role to play in its contemporary management).

Blastocyst Embryo Stage Transfer (BEST)

In routine IVF treatment the embryo is transferred into the womb about 48 hours old, usually a 2–4 cell structure by now, which in spontaneous pregnancy would still be in the Fallopian tube. With blastocyst transfer, embryo transfer is delayed until 5 or 6 days after fertilisation when the embryo might comprise up to 100 cells already. This has the advantages that the embryo is transferred to the womb at the same time as it would get there spontaneously, and that the most viable embryos can be selected.

Whilst this technique is over 16 years old, it has taken many years to develop the right culture medium with the right balance of nutrients to sustain embryo growth outside the womb. CARE in Nottingham are pioneers in this technique in the UK. Of the 48 patients they have treated, results proved a higher pregnancy success rate with blastocyst transfers than conventional transfers (50 per cent compared to 42 per cent) but this has to be compared in turn to the fact that there is between 70–40 per cent risk of loss of embryos in extended culture and that therefore not all patients might be suitable candidates.

Pre-Implantation Genetic Diagnosis (Embryo Screening) or PGD
This highly controversial technique is an IVF procedure, with the added
stage of screening out potentially fatal genetic diseases at embryo stage
before transfer to the womb. Some hereditary disorders such as haemophilia,
Duchenne muscular dystrophy and certain mental and physical disabilities
are 'sex-linked', that is, only carried by one gender. Others could be carried
by either sex. Rare single-gene-defect conditions such as Tay Sachs disease
(which causes death in infancy) have been screened, as well as thalassaemia
(a form of anaemia) and cystic fibrosis, whilst research into screening for
Down Syndrome, cancer (15 genes for inherited cancer have been identified)
and chromosome disorders leading to recurrent miscarriage continues.

Some pundits say that this technique could virtually eliminate certain
diseases. It provokes enormous anxiety and ethical questions about doctors
playing God. Screening (by sex-selection in some cases) and preventing the
births of children with impairments is in effect genetic engineering and will
inevitably continue to raise a great deal of controversy. But for desperate
couples with the misfortune of a fatal genetic disease in the family, it is a
choice offered by the revolution in reproductive science.

Embryo screening, like selective termination, occupies an extremely
thorny terrain in the ART landscape. Genetic selection frightens because it
evokes eugenics. Understandably the disabled community have strong views
on the subject (*see Issues, pages 206–230*).

Pre-implantation diagnosis follows the same procedure as IVF, with
hormonally-stimulated egg production followed by egg collection. About
48–72 hours after fertilisation, a single cell is extracted from each embryo,
which is then biochemically examined and DNA-tested for the presence of
the defective gene. If this results in a suspected defect, the biopsied cell is
subjected to further tests. If not, the embryo(s) will be transferred into the
womb as per normal IVF.

WHAT ARE THE RISKS ASSOCIATED WITH EMBRYO SCREENING?
There are the risks associated with routine IVF to consider (multiple births,
failure to produce a pregnancy) plus a possible increased risk of miscarriage
and a slight chance that the diagnosis itself might be incorrect. Other than
that, there is currently no evidence of the technique causing damage to the
embryo itself. However, as with all the newest methods, experts advise
regular medical assessments of any child born. Pre-implantation diagnosis is
a sophisticated branch of ART research and development, and still at a very
early stage of experimentation.

Egg Donation

Where a woman is not producing eggs (because of an early menopause, as a result of chemotherapy, ovarian disease, age, etc.) she may be eligible for egg donation. Egg donation is another branch of ART developed through IVF research. Essentially it involves fertilising donor eggs with the recipient man's sperm, freezing the resulting embryo(s), preparing the recipient and transferring the thawed embryos into the woman's uterus. Many couples opt for this since at least the baby born would be genetically half their own and the pregnancy allows the couple to bond with the baby. Since it is often the case that the woman who isn't producing eggs may also not be producing the right level of reproductive hormones, she may be given oestrogen prior to embryo transfer to encourage implantation. The egg donor can be anonymous or known (such as a family member). The donor will have to go through an IVF treatment cycle up to and including egg collection.

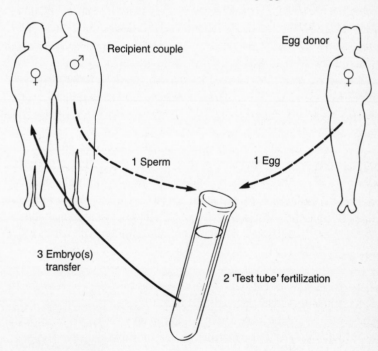

1. Sperm from recipient
   egg from donor ovary

3. Embryo(s) to recipient womb

Figure 19: Egg donation.

The recipient woman's cycle may be manipulated into synchrony with the donor's, or embryos may be frozen and replaced at a later date.

Donated eggs must be used 'fresh' to create embryos since, unlike sperm, it isn't possible to freeze them. Egg donors therefore have to undergo ovarian stimulation and egg collection. This may be a factor in why it is hard to access potential donors and why there are such long waiting lists. The Lister Hospital in London reported in July 1996 that it had 700 women waiting for donor eggs. Egg shortages are a problem in the UK, particularly eggs from women of certain ethnic minorities. However, the success of recent egg donation campaigns have proven that it is also a simple problem of public ignorance. NURTURE in Nottingham solved their egg shortage problem within a matter of days after a media-assisted egg-donor campaign. And King's Assisted Conception Unit recently launched a very high-profile egg-donation campaign to educate the public and encourage donors to come forward.

Screening of the donor is crucial. The donor will also be screened for viral infections such as hepatitis, HIV, etc. and possibly undergo genetic screening. The egg donor is required by law to disclose any inherited disease which may result in the birth of a disabled baby.

Egg donation cycles are more successful than routine IVF, probably because the eggs are from young women (the donor age limit is 35) and also because the woman recipient won't have undergone superovulation drug treatment which, ironically, can produce far too much oestrogen which can cause the lining of the womb to become too thick to allow implantation. Thus her womb will be in a 'natural' state of receptivity. Many clinics will treat women over the age of 45 with donor eggs (*see 'A User's Guide', page 245*).

EGG DONORS
These women may be related to the couple or anonymous. Where they are anonymous, they would be matched as far as possible in race and type to the woman recipient. Anonymous egg donors may be women who are themselves going through IVF, GIFT, or any treatment in which a surplus of eggs may be produced through hormone treatment. They may occasionally be women who want to help other women and go through the whole operation purely altruistically.

Tess: I can tell you what I do every single day. I walk down the street and leer at women. Which one has the good eggs? There's an exhausted twenty-year-old with three brutalised children. Shall I tell her I'll get her out of her rut in exchange for her eggs – but what kind of genes does she have? I spot a young mother in a book store, perfect: brainy eggs. She goes to the feminist section, she'll wonder why my only identity is motherhood. There's a foreign student. I fantasise about kidnapping her. I wouldn't have pity. I sit on a park bench like a flasher. Women used to be my sisters. They're objects: egg vessels. Now you know.

TIMBERLAKE WERTENBAKER, *BREAK OF DAY* (FABER & FABER, 1996)

ANONYMITY

The HF & E Act of 1990 stipulates the following as regards the identity of donors: by law the donor relinquishes all legal rights and claims over any offspring which they may have helped create. Conversely, the donor's identity will by law remain anonymous. However, non-identifying information about the donor such as hair colour, nationality and height must be registered with the HFEA. The donor can, if they wish, also provide information on their interests and occupation. Any child born by gamete donation has legal right of access to this non-identifying information at the age of 18 years. For a fuller discussion of the issues of family and genetic origin, please refer to Chapter 7.

Egg Sharing

This is a new development in the UK, although egg sharing has been going on in other countries for some years. In 1992 at least 45 per cent of US clinics offered egg sharing, whilst in Israel egg sharing is the only legal form of donation.

Now hospitals such as the Cromwell in London run 'egg sharing schemes' where a woman undergoing IVF agrees to donate half her eggs per treatment cycle in exchange for a free treatment (although the couple still has to pay certain expenses, such as for first consultation, semen analysis and blood tests). It has proved very successful.

A pilot study at the Cromwell Hospital was reported in the journal *Human Reproduction* in 1996. Interestingly it showed that whilst the recipients were older than the donors (egg donors must be under 35), the success rates amongst recipients was 30 per cent as opposed to 20 per cent amongst donors. This proved that age-related decline in fertility is indeed associated with egg quality and quantity rather than with the uterus (about

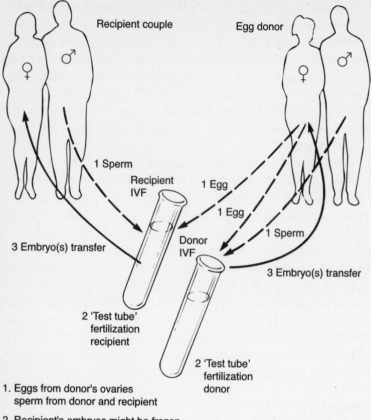

1. Eggs from donor's ovaries
   sperm from donor and recipient

2. Recipient's embryos might be frozen
   and transferred to womb later

3. Embryo(s) transferred to wombs

Figure 20: Egg sharing.

which the profession still actually know little). The report concluded that egg sharing is a very 'constructive' way of solving the current shortage of donor eggs, but that:

The ideal of pure altruism is not without its medical and moral risk. The success of egg-sharing depends on shared interests and a degree of altruism between the donor, the recipient and the centre.

HUMAN REPRODUCTION VOL. 11, NO 5 (1996): PAGES 1126–31

Women who choose to donate their eggs tend to be proud and happy that they can help other women in this way. A woman on GLR's Jewish London edition, speaking on infertility in June 1996, told listeners how delighted she had been at each of her (eight!) donation cycles at the Lister Hospital.

The HFEA conducted a survey in 1993 into the motivations and attitudes of sperm and egg donors. Male donors were concerned about being contacted by offspring, and admitted that both a desire to help others and payment influenced their decision to become donors. Women, on the other hand, were all motivated by a wish to help others rather than payment and were more concerned than men about the possible existence of children they would never know.

EGG DONATION AND COUNSELLING
Because of the emotional, social, medical and ethical issues involved, both recipients and donors by law should be given careful counselling to ensure that both parties fully understand the implications of this form of treatment.

PAYMENT TO EGG DONORS
See pages 224–5.

Donor Embryos
Donated embryos might be donated at the time they are created as part of an IVF cycle, or, more often, donated after embryo freezing when the donor(s) would have achieved a successful pregnancy. Donor embryos might be used when, for example, a woman has for whatever reasons ceased egg production. Evidence suggests that the age of the womb might have less influence on achieving pregnancy than the deterioration of egg quality and production with age. In a donor embryo cycle, monitoring and/or manipulating the correct production of hormones for the recipient are distinct procedures from that concerning the donor who will have undergone an IVF cycle to produce surplus embryos. The recipient's womb lining must be able to receive the embryos for implantation. She might reach this in a natural cycle, in which case she would be monitored by ultrasound for the optimum time to carry out embryo transfer. Or, where she may need hormonal stimulation, she would be given HRT (hormonal replacement therapy) which she would continue taking until she is 3 months pregnant, after which the placenta should take over normal hormone production for the development of the foetus.

Although embryo donation has become a relatively straightforward procedure, it brings with it social, emotional and ethical problems which need to be resolved before embarking on a treatment cycle so as not to be overwhelmed with it later.

MR ANDREW KAN AND MR HOSSAM ABDULLA, THE LISTER HOSPITAL: *CHILD FACTSHEET*

Embryo Freezing/Cryopreservation

Since the HF & E Act of 1990, a maximum of three embryos are allowed to be transferred to the uterus in any one treatment cycle. Superovulation drugs can stimulate the ovaries to produce as many as 20 eggs in one cycle, many of which might fertilise. Embryo freezing allows for spare embryos to be stored for later use (for example, where a treatment fails or when the couple want a second child/more children) thus bypassing another cycle of intensive drug stimulation, egg and sperm collection and fertilisation.

Since the first human child was born from a frozen embryo in Australia in 1984, cryopreservation has become common practice in IVF clinics.

WHEN IS EMBRYO FREEZING ADVISED?

Some people feel extremely uncomfortable about wasting embryos, and may choose to freeze their spares for their own or other people's use or in the interests of research. It might also be recommended to women over 40 whose egg production is in danger of sudden deterioration. If a woman falls ill (as with ovarian hyperstimulation) during a treatment cycle, making embryo transfer impossible, freezing can be a real advantage. A woman who knows she is to undergo cancer treatment causing sterility can opt to have embryos frozen for future use should she survive her illness.

The advantage of using frozen embryos is that it is much cheaper and less invasive than IVF from scratch. Most IVF clinics now have storage facilities and it is largely considered a routine practice.

The technique of embryo freezing is complex. Fluid is removed from the embryonic cells by treating them with a chemical 'antifreeze', and the dehydrated cell structure is put in a straw together with a cryoprotectant solution, frozen and stored in liquid nitrogen at a temperature of minus 190° Fahrenheit. The thawing process involves slowly replacing the cryoprotectant with water.

Embryo Transfer (ET)

Transfer of frozen embryos is similar to an insemination treatment. Embryos may be replaced in synchrony with the woman's natural cycle or ovulation may be suppressed and the uterine lining prepared. Then a suppressant drug will be prescribed to cease your own egg production during this cycle. This would be followed by oestrogen, whilst your hormone levels will be monitored with scans and blood tests to check for the condition of the uterine lining. Progesterone is given before embryo transfer, which would be via the cervix with a catheter. Generally speaking, the success rate in terms of live births using frozen embryos is not as high as with 'fresh' embryos (12.7 per cent as compared to 14.7 per cent).

RISKS OF EMBRYO FREEZING

Cryopreservation undoubtedly causes shock to the embryos, whilst the long-term effects are still unknown and are the subject of some debate. What is known is that the chemicals used in the freeze/thaw process are 'quite toxic' (Professor Winston). In fact, many embryos don't survive the thawing process, whilst there is evidence of damage to those that do. Cryopreservation kills off a number of cells, and in thawed embryos the DNA structure sometimes appears to have been disrupted. A recent French experiment conducted on mice embryos did show abnormalities in later life, including obesity, alterations to the jaw and behavioural abnormalities. Professor Winston uses this evidence to remain extremely 'cautious' about the long-term risks of cryopreservation. He is concerned about the risk of leukaemia and infertility in babies born from frozen embryos. He tends to stand alone on this. Many specialists strongly disagree with his position and feel confident about the process or, as Dr Simon Fishel says, as confident as one might be of any of the processes of IVF.

Cryopreservation is a relatively new technique and we can't possibly know the long-term effects yet. Thus, like with so many of ART's offerings, we must take responsibility for our own participation in the long-term experiment of it all. To give you an idea of the scale of cryopreservation, in the summer of 1995 52,000 embryos were in storage in the UK. In September 2000, the journal *Progress in Reproduction* (Vol. 4), reported that 250,000 embryos have been stored in the UK.

FOR HOW LONG CAN EMBRYOS BE STORED?

The HF & E Act in 1990 legislated for five years. This frustrated many specialists, who argued that this was an arbitrary length of time. Professional pressure has been put on the HFEA to extend this to 10 years (or more in certain cases); these new regulations came into effect on 1st May 1996. Any parents with embryos frozen between August 1991 and May 1996 could apply for an extension. In fact thousands of unclaimed 'orphan' embryos were destroyed on 1st August 1996 because clinics were unable to trace their parents. The whole issue provoked intense media coverage and, inevitably, huge outcry from the Pro-Life camp, who demanded that the State 'adopt' these 'orphans'. The HFEA meanwhile held firm to their commitment to the law, which states that genetic material belongs to the parents and not the State. In fact, clinics are given guardianship over frozen genetic matter and in the 'Big Thaw' were acting as such. One tragedy of the waste was that the profession could have used them for research.

The problem of 'neglected' frozen embryos continues. In April 2000 the *Lancet* reported that in two of Britain's fertility clinics two-thirds of embryos had to be destroyed because of the HFEA 5 year rule. The authors speculate that the reasons for the waste might be economic. A high proportion of couples contacted didn't respond, whilst a significant proportion of those who did were NHS patients, suggesting that cost might be a deterrent in couples requesting an extended storage time.

REPORTED IN THE *GUARDIAN* 14TH APRIL 2000

Sperm Freezing

This technique has been used in cattle breeding for many years and on evidence is entirely safe. Sperm is cultured for infection and all donor sperm is screened for HIV. Frozen sperm, whilst widely used in ART, tends to be less fertile than fresh sperm, with reduced motility and endurance once put inside the woman's reproductive system.

Apart from donor sperm and some of the ART techniques mentioned above, sperm freezing can be used when the man knows he is going to have treatment for cancer. His sperm can be stored until he wishes to use it to make a baby in the future. It may also be stored prior to an ART cycle if problems are anticipated with producing sperm samples 'to order'.

Egg Freezing

This is one of the latest procedures to be licensed in the UK. Women in Britain have been free to freeze their eggs since 1998. But in January 2000 the HFEA granted the first licence to a UK clinic – the Assisted Reproduction and Gynaecology Centre in London – to thaw human eggs. CARE at The Park offers egg freezing to patients who are at risk of becoming infertile from cancer treatment. Egg-freezing follows the same procedure as IVF in terms of drug-stimulated super-ovulation and egg-collection. The eggs are then stored in liquid nitrogen for up to ten years. The *Times* newspaper reported in March 2000 that it is expected that many more clinics will be applying to the HFEA in the near future and that Britain is 'on the verge of a frozen baby boom'.

I am self-employed and I do not have the time or the money for children ... That's why I will consider having my eggs frozen – I regard children as a serious commitment, not a fashion accessory.
DEA PARKIN, QUOTED IN THE *DAILY MAIL*, 2ND FEBRUARY 2000

Ovarian Tissue Freezing

This is one of the most recent advances in fertility techniques. It has been found that microscopic pieces of ovarian tissue can be frozen, thawed and then cultured to produce eggs. So far experts have only managed to grow eggs to the first stage of maturation, but are confident that the technique will be perfected within 5–10 years' time. This technique could revolutionise IVF treatment in the future. A woman could have her potential eggs stored when she is young for use when she is older, bypassing the need for drug treatment to stimulate ovulation.

Last October I froze the ovaries of a 3-year-old-girl. They will remain on ice, at the taxpayer's expense, until she is old enough to have children ... My motivations were simple; without this intervention she would have become sterile.
PROFESSOR ROGER GOSDEN OF LEEDS UNIVERSITY ON A PATIENT UNDERGOING RADIATION FOR A TUMOUR ON HER KIDNEY, AS REPORTED IN THE *DAILY EXPRESS*, 19TH MARCH 1996

In 1994 the HFEA held a consultation on the sensitive issues surrounding the use of donated ovarian tissue in embryo research and infertility treatment. At the time debate was rife as to whether ovarian tissue should be extracted from cadavers and foetuses, and the press had a field day with sensationalist headlines about using aborted material to create babies. The HFEA concluded that ovarian tissue could be used only from live donors. (*See pages 221–3 for a fuller discussion of these issues.*)

In Vitro Maturation

This is a process whereby the egg is collected whilst still immature from the ovary and matured *in vitro* to the point where it is ripe for fertilisation. This can be done either with or without ovarian drug stimulation.

Surrogacy

And when Rachel saw that she bore Jacob no children, Rachel envied her sister; and said unto Jacob, Give me children else I die.

And Jacob's anger was kindled against Rachel; and he said, Am I in God's stead, who hath withheld from thee the fruit of the womb?

And she said, Behold my maid Bilbah, go unto her; and she shall bear upon my knees, that I may also have children by her.[5]

GENESIS 30:1–3

Surrogacy is a last option for infertile people, since it is a lengthy, hazardous and psychologically demanding route to a child of your own. Surrogacy itself doesn't fall within the remit of the HFEA (although the IVF procedure involved does) but is covered by the Department of Health under the Surrogacy Arrangements Act of 1985.

In February 1996 the British Medical Association changed its own policy towards surrogacy and declared it acceptable. The BMA had originally been advising doctors to have nothing to do with surrogacy. When it later told doctors they could help, it then added the proviso that the two parties should have as little to do with each other as possible, for fear of psychological problems. Now, the BMA in conjunction with the HFEA have produced a booklet entitled 'Considering Surrogacy? Your questions answered' in which, amongst other issues covered, the benefits of both parties supporting each other through the process are asserted.

With surrogacy, a third party (woman) carries and delivers a baby for an infertile couple. There are two types of surrogacy, the first using insemination and the second by IVF:

Straight surrogacy

(also known as 'traditional' or 'partial'):
The surrogate artificially inseminates herself with the husband's sperm (this can also be done by a health professional).

Host surrogacy

(also known as 'full' or 'IVF'):
The surrogate has no genetic involvement in the embryo but acts as an 'incubator'. The couple's embryos, formed through IVF, are transferred into the surrogate.

STRAIGHT SURROGACY

Whilst technically speaking this could be done by any consenting adults with no medical intervention prior to pregnancy, it is highly recommended that all parties concerned have full tests for HIV, hepatitis and possibly genetic screening. Some Family Health Practices will carry out these checks for free, but results may take time. Private hospitals offer the full tests for fees of around £100 to £250.

Once the surrogate has agreed, the procedure is the same as for insemination, with all the potential for failure at first and the possible need for several attempts. This means that the man has to produce sperm and deliver it to the surrogate on a frequent basis until a pregnancy has been achieved. The surrogate then proceeds with routine antenatal care at her local hospital. The commissioning couple may be able to be present at the birth, depending on agreements established with the surrogate and the hospital itself.

HOST SURROGACY

This can only be undertaken under medical supervision at an IVF clinic. The commissioning woman will undergo a complete IVF treatment cycle up to and including egg collection, whilst the man produces fresh sperm on that same day. Any fertilised embryos may be frozen for six months for full HIV screening, or transferred to the host immediately if full HIV screening has taken place to the satisfaction of the HFEA stipulations.

The surrogate then has the embryos transferred into her uterus in the same way as any frozen embryo transfer. However, some clinics prefer to medicalise the process by suppressing the host's natural cycle with hormone treatment. The rationale for this is to ensure that the surrogate can't become pregnant by other means during the surrogacy attempt.

HIV and Other Tests

The HFEA has no jurisdiction over surrogacy itself, but all its laws and regulations regarding IVF, DI and donor gametes apply to surrogacy:

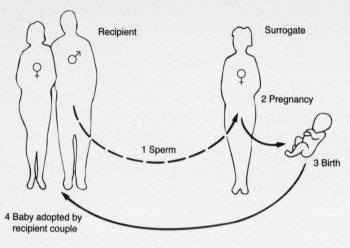

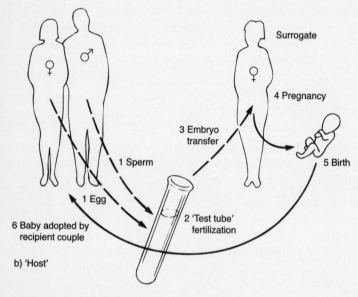

a) 'Straight'

b) 'Host'

1. Recipient egg and sperm
2. IVF
3. Embryo(s) transferred to surrogate's womb
4. Surrogate gestates baby/babies
5. Surrogate gives birth
6. Surrogate gives up baby/babies for adoption
   by recipient couple

Figure 21: Surrogacy. a) 'Straight'. b) 'Host'.

As with all organs and tissues for transplantation donors of gametes (semen and eggs) must be shown to be free of infection with HIV. This entails testing the blood of donors for HIV antibody at the time donations are made.
HFEA CODE OF PRACTICE, REVISED EDITION DECEMBER 1995; ANNEX C, PAGE 61

Since antibodies sometimes don't appear for up to six months after infection, HIV screening involves a period of quarantine. Normally this would be done by blood testing both man and woman before the eggs and sperm are taken, freezing the resulting embryos for six months, and repeating the HIV tests on both parties and only transferring the embryo(s) to the surrogate if these tests are negative.

Some clinics don't have the facilities for embryo freezing, in which case the semen would be stored and the man tested for HIV both prior to this and six months later, whilst the woman would be blood-tested at assessment stage and at egg collection, carrying only a very 'small risk' of infection which should be fully explained to all parties.

SURROGACY AND THE LAW
Surrogacy itself is controlled by the Surrogacy Arrangements Act of 1985, whilst the use of gametes, DI and IVF are under the control of the HFEA.

Who Is the Legal Parent of a Child Born by Surrogacy?
This is one of the hardest and most hazardous aspects of surrogacy. By law the commissioning father is the legal father and the surrogate the legal mother. This means that in order for the child or children born to become legally both parents', the commissioning couple have to adopt them.
The legal implications of this are quite treacherous to all parties concerned. The surrogate has the legal right to change her mind about handing over the baby at birth, even if the baby she is carrying isn't genetically hers. Conversely, the commissioning parents might change their minds during the surrogate's pregnancy, in which case the surrogate becomes legally responsible for the offspring. Mutual trust is therefore absolutely essential between all parties concerned.

SURROGACY AND MONEY
The Surrogacy Arrangements Act forbids any commercial transactions between commissioning couples and surrogates. 'Expenses' may be paid by mutual arrangement and these can run into thousands of pounds, covering antenatal care, work interruption for the surrogate and her medical

expenses. Clearly legislation over financial dealings is desirable. Without it the spectre of ruthless agencies exploiting impoverished women willing to rent out their wombs at risk of mental and physical health looms large and real in the present economy.

THE EMOTIONAL AND SOCIAL IMPLICATIONS OF SURROGACY

These are vast and complex and finally can only be resolved by the parties concerned. The surrogate needs to be sure of her own motivation, the support she may or may not get from friends and family, the realities of giving birth and, crucially, the separation from the baby born. The commissioning couple and surrogate need to explore together key issues such as their views on amniocentesis tests for chromosome abnormalities and how much contact they wish to maintain both during the pregnancy and afterwards, with particular consideration of the welfare of the eventual child(ren) born. The commissioning couple need to ensure that their motivation, support (mutual and from outside the relationship), emotional and ethical issues have been aired and agreed.

C.O.T.S. (CHILDLESSNESS OVERCOME THROUGH SURROGACY)

This charity was founded by Kim Cotton (who caused bitter furore in 1985 when she gave birth for £6,500 for a childless American couple) and Gena Dodd, reputedly the first mother in the UK to have used a surrogate to carry her son in 1984.

C.O.T.S. devotes itself to help, advise and support both infertile couples and surrogates as well as aiming to enhance public awareness about surrogacy. They work in close contact with IVF Hospitals involved in host surrogacy and can put people in touch with psychologists, counsellors and solicitors specialising in the subject.

C.O.T.S. itself can't actually advertise for surrogates but must wait for potential surrogates to approach them. They have a carefully constructed contact procedure by which couples and surrogates can choose to meet. Members of C.O.T.S., once seen by a mediator/counsellor, automatically become members of Triangle, a splinter group of C.O.T.S. Triangle then compiles a list of infertile couples (excluding their name and address) with details about their physical type, reasons for infertility, age and profession. The surrogate chooses a couple(s) off the list she may wish to help and is then sent their 'details'. If she wishes to proceed, the couple are sent her 'details'. If all parties still wish to meet they are supplied with names and addresses.

II Drugs

A priory

Discreet containers
catch urine from
the ageing nuns.
Strange potion for
seeds of life.
ANONYMOUS (EXTRACT FROM 'SCENES FROM INFERTILITY',
PROSPECT NEWSLETTER NO 31, SPRING 1996)

This poem is musing on the strange provenance of, until very recently, one
of the key ingredients used in fertility drugs: human female, post-
menopausal urine. In the early days of fertility drugs one cycle of fertility
treatment could require as much as 30 litres of the stuff. Serono, one of the
world's largest infertility drug manufacturing companies, reported in 1995
receiving 40,000 gallons of urine per day, collected by road tanker, mostly
but not exclusively from Italian nuns. It's an awesome thought.

The problem with urine-derived preparations is that they contain
unwanted impurities and proteins which can cause allergic reactions.
Furthermore, administering these drugs can be quite painful as they have
to be injected directly into the buttock in large quantities, and necessitate
daily visits to a clinic. Today, whilst urine is still used in some fertility drugs,
manufacturing extraction techniques have developed versions which are far

purer. The real advantage of these new products is that they can be injected subcutaneously (directly under the skin). Furthermore, the injection is comparatively tiny in volume and simple enough for self-administration.

Clearly this is hugely beneficial as it empowers the woman and avoids the hassle of early morning trips to the professionals. Today, an increasing number of women are offered the choice to administer their own fertility drugs. Your clinic should offer you a demonstration prior to this procedure. There is even a free Home Care Plan which delivers all drugs and equipment directly to the patient's home at an agreed time of day in unmarked packaging for discretion.

For those who feel anxious about using syringes and needles, you will be relieved to know that there are new and very convenient, relatively pain-free gadgets on the market. The first of these is the Auto-injector. This is spring-loaded and both the drug dose and needle are delivered at the touch of a button so that you don't have to go through the ordeal of pushing a needle into your own skin. The second, and faster to administer, is the Fertility Pen. Similar to that used by diabetics, this is loaded with a multidose cartridge which you assemble yourself. Your individually prescribed dose is then dialed and instantly released. The huge advantage of this device is that you can take your 'pen' away for a few days, loaded up with enough doses you need for that time, liberating you from what used to be the phase in a treatment cycle when your endurance would be tested by a strict regime full of bruising injection appointments at your clinic. Both of these options are convenient, easy to use and reduce local pain and irritation, which is why currently 80% are self-injecting at home in the UK.

Whilst manufacturers and doctors prescribing these drugs assure us of their safety, it is worth knowing as much as possible about them, what they are composed of, what they do and any possible side-effects. Fertility drugs are powerful substances which adjust your entire reproductive hormone balance. There is no getting away from the fact that they are likely to have some side-effects, but these will obviously vary from person to person. Remember, patient information must be supplied by the manufacturer and you should read this small print carefully. Don't be afraid to ask questions at the clinic about the drugs you are prescribed. If you aren't reacting well or are allergic there may be alternatives – different brands or dosages. It's your body, so don't suffer its abuse in silence.

There are four main drugs involved in infertility treatment, though not all of them will be used in any one fertility clinic:[v]

1. Drugs which SUPPRESS your natural menstrual cycle
2. Drugs which STIMULATE your ovaries to ripen follicles
3. Drugs which CAUSE OVULATION
4. Drugs which SUPPORT embryo implantation.

Basically, what fertility drugs do is manipulate your natural ovarian production via a procedure whereby a blank canvas is created by suppressing ovulation (effectively giving you a temporary menopause) known as 'down-regulation'. Once this has been achieved, this is reversed by ovarian stimulation so that, hopefully, you super-ovulate, producing sometimes as many as 20 or more eggs in one go. This, as a recent article in *CHILDchat* (Autumn 2000 Edition no 89) by Richard Fleming of the ACS Unit at Glasgow Royal Infirmary explains, is because the clinic needs to 'be able to control ovarian function without interference'.

In this article Fleming goes on to explain another recent breakthrough in fertility drugs: the use of what are known as GnHR antagonists. As we have seen earlier in the book, the ovaries are controlled by two hormones, the gonadotrophins FSH (follicle stimulating hormone) and LH, luteinising hormone. These are in turn controlled by a single hormone GnRH. Once the structure of this hormone was established, chemists were able to develop different drugs (called GnRH analogs) which, by mimicking these hormones, trigger the body's own over or underproduction of the LH or FSH hormones resulting in either the suppression of or stimulation of ovulation. This is because once the structure of the GnRH was known, researchers were able to make different versions of it which are known as *agonists* or *antagonists*. Agonists stimulate FSH and LH output in the short term, but after prolonged use reverse this and become a suppressor. These are the drugs in the first category listed overleaf and are usually sniffed during the first phase of a treatment cycle. GnHr antagonists on the contrary were found to block the release of LH and FSH with immediate effect . Recently new versions of these antagonists have been developed which act very rapidly with minimum side-effect. It is these drugs that Fleming calls 'the new kid on the block' and which he advocates as a serious breakthrough since 'we do not require the down regulation pre-treatment and can administer the drug after we have started to stimulate the ovaries. This makes the whole treatment cycle shorter ... With the down-regulation induced by the GnHR analogs, some patients have to endure unpleasant side-effects of menopausal symptoms. This problem will be eliminated by the antagonists'. Finally, another possible pro of the increased availability and use of the antagonists is that they may reduce the risk of OHSS (ovarian hyperstimulation syndrome) and that poor responders may respond better to them. However, such suggestions cannot be confirmed until further clinical trials are carried out.

The following is meant as a guide to the kinds of drugs you might currently meet in your treatment. It isn't by any means exhaustive as there are a lot of fertility drugs on the market.

NB: **Not everyone experiences side-effects to the same degree, and some may hardly feel any symptoms at all. The information below is an indication of what the drugs are known to have caused a proportion of women.**

1. Suppressing Drugs

a) Agonist:

Brands (examples):	Buserelin, Nafarelin, Zoladex, Signarel
Used to:	Block LH surge so that ovulation is (temporarily) stopped
In which treatments:	IVF/GIFT/Surrogacy/Frozen Embryo Transfer (ET)
How it works:	Stimulates the pituitary gland and then de-sensitises it so that FSH and LH levels from the pituitary drop
Administered by:	Nasal spray or injection
Side-effects:	The drug simulates menopause; symptoms can include hot flushes and sweats, mood swings, irregular bleeding, vaginal dryness, 'head cold'
Risks/contra-indications:	Not to be used where there is a pituitary dysfunction or risk of osteoporosis. Not to be used in conjuntion with hormonal methods of birth control, when pregnant or lactating

b) Antagonist:

Brands (examples):	Cetrotide, Orgalutron
Used to:	Prevent premature ovulation
In which treatments:	Controlled ovarian stimulation (IVF and associated techniques)
How it works:	Prevents the premature LH surge
Administered by:	Injection (subcutaneous)
Side-effects:	Nausea, headaches
Risks/contra-indications:	Not to be used during post-menopause, pregnancy or where there is renal or hepatic impairment

2. Ovary-stimulating Drugs

a) Anti-oestrogens:

Brands (examples):	Serophene/Clomid or Tamoxifen (Nolvadex)
Used to:	Trigger pituitary hormones to stimulate ovaries
In which treatments:	Ovulatory disorders (such as long cycles, irregular periods)/DI
How it works:	Mimics oestrogen and 'fools' the brain into absorbing it instead, so that the brain consequently misreads oestrogen levels and activates natural release of FSH from pituitary, leading to ovulation
Administered by:	Tablets
Side-effects:	Hot flushes, mood swings, depression, nausea, breast tenderness. (*NB*: drug should be immediately stopped if headaches and/or visual disturbance occur) nervousness, insomnia, increased urination, heavy periods, fatigue, skin reaction, weight gain. Can cause cervical mucus thickening, preventing sperm from swimming up cervical canal
Risks/contra-indications:	Not to be used where there is liver disease or dysfunction, ovarian cysts (other than due to Polycystic Ovarian Syndrome), ovarian endometriosis. Can cause multiple pregnancy

b) hMG (Human Menopausal Gonadotrophin)

Brands (examples):	Menogon, Menopure
Used to:	Stimulate the ovary to ripen follicles, assist sperm production
In which treatments:	Anovulation, and for controlled superovulation in IVF, GIFT, ZIFT, IUI and when there is deficient sperm development due to poor pituitary function
How it works:	Drug contains the pituitary hormones FSH, which stimulates egg maturation, and LH, which stimulates egg release. In the male LH and FSH stimulate sperm development and testosterone production
Administered by:	Injection (intra-muscular)
Side-effects:	Breast tenderness, abdominal bloating, mood swings, aching muscles and joints, allergic reactions such as rashes, pain or bruising at injection site, and fever
Risks/contra-indications:	Ovarian hyperstimulation, multiple pregnancies, miscarriage. Should not be used by pregnant or lactating women, nor where there are ovarian, testicular or pituitary tumours

c) FSH (Follicle Stimulating Hormone)

Brands (examples):	Metrodin High Purity, Gonal-F, Puragon
Used to:	Stimulate ovulation
In which treatments:	Anovulation, controlled superovulation (IVF, GIFT, ZIFT, IUI), assumed to be advantageous to women with Polycystic Ovarian Syndrome who have high LH level
How it works:	Contains almost no LH, otherwise it is identical to hMG
Administered by:	Injection (subcutaneous)
Side-effects:	Abdominal bloating, mood swings, rashes, painful muscles and joints, allergic reactions at injection site such as rashes (but less common than with hMG), bruising, fever

Risks/contra-indications: Multiple pregnancy, ovarian hyperstimulation, miscarriage. Not to be used if pregnant, where there is cancer of breast, ovaries, uterus, fibroid tumours in uterus

d) LHRH (Luteinising Hormone Releasing Hormone)

Brand (example):   Fertiral

Used to: Stimulate the ovary

In which treatments: Anovulation (where pituitary hormone levels are low), superovulation (as an alternative to gonadotrophins)

How it works: Restores LHRH level by mimicking its natural secretion – 'pulses' occurring approximately every 90 minutes.

Administered by: Infusion pump worn night and day (for example under the arm) which automatically injects hormone under the skin at regular intervals

Side-effects: Has advantage over hMG as this treatment stimulates an almost-natural cycle with no hyperstimulation and no multiple pregnancies

Risks, contra-indications: Can cause abdominal pain, nausea, headaches, excessive menstual bleeding. Should not be taken where there are endometriotic cysts, PCOS, weight-related amenhorrhoea before correction of weight loss. Should not be taken following conception or for more than 6 months

e) Bromocriptine

Brand (example):   Parlodel

Used to: Stimulate ovulation by reducing prolactin level

In which treatments: Ovulation disorders associated with high prolactinconception or after 6 months levels

How it works: 20 per cent of women have irregular or no periods because they produce too much prolactin. This drug rapidly lowers prolactin level

Administered by: Tablets
Side-effects: Dizziness, headaches, nausea, lassitude

3. Drugs to Trigger Ovulation

hCG (Human Chorionic Gonadotrophin)

Brands (examples):   Pregnyl, Profasi
Used to: Trigger ovulation in women and to improve
                          sperm development in men
In which treatments: Anovulation, absence of follicle rupture and
                          with controlled superovulation (IVF, GIFT,
                          ZIFT, IUI)
How it works: hCG is a hormone produced by early embryo
                          and placenta, identical to LH in its action.
                          It is given prior to the time of expected LH
                          surge to trigger ovulation (in controlled
                          superovulation as 'midnight injection' prior
                          to egg collection). In men, helps testicles
                          produce testosterone
Administered by: Injection
Side-effects: Skin rashes, water retention (in men)
Risks/contra-indications: Can produce ovarian hyperstimulation,
                          multiple births, miscarriage. Not to be used
                          where there are known or suspected cancers
                          (in men) and to be used with caution and
                          monitoring where there is cardiac failure,
                          renal dysfunction, hypertension, epilepsy
                          or migraine

4. Drugs that Support Pregnancy Following ART Treatment

a) Progesterone

Brands (examples):   Cyclogest, Crinone
Used to: Boost body's natural progesterone production
In which treatment: Following embryo transfer in Assisted
                          Conception

How it works:	Enhances body's own production to help the cells of the endometrium (womb lining) thicken to assist implantation, build protein and store sugar in preparation to nurture the embryo
Administered by:	Injections, pessaries
Side-effects:	'Pregnancy symptoms' such as nausea, swollen breasts. Injections can cause bruising of muscle tissue and soreness
Risks, contra-indications:	Undiagnosed vaginal bleeding, liver dysfunction

b) hCG Injections

As above.

Antibiotics

Both the man (before giving the sperm sample that will be used in fertilisation) and the woman may be prescribed antibiotics to prevent any infection from interfering with IVF treatments.

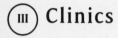 # Clinics

Why the Expanding ART Market?

Provision of IVF treatment in the UK has greatly increased since 1978. Clinics seem to have been springing up like mushrooms so that now there are well over 100 units of varying sizes and expertise. Some of them are exclusively NHS but most are operating a 'mixed economy', whilst many remain exclusively private.

It is doubtful whether anyone then appreciated the enormous commercial potential of their work. It has transformed both the profit and loss account and the balance sheet of gynaecology beyond recognition. Shortly after the birth of the first 'test-tube baby', increasing numbers of gynaecologists began to treat involuntarily childless women using assisted conception techniques.
NAOMI PFEFFER, *THE STORK AND THE SYRINGE* (POLITY PRESS, 1993)

Some private doctors are shamelessly lining their pockets from the profits of desperation. Other consultants such as Lord Professor Winston of the Hammersmith Hospital have found 'Robin Hood' solutions to the lack of national NHS funding: in a strategy for some kind of redistribution of wealth, the Hammersmith siphons off its profits from private practice and puts them into research projects.

The trouble with running a Health Service like a big corporation is that a competitive market is created in which hospitals compete with each other

for money, patients and – in the case of fertility treatment – licenses.
On paper it may look great that there is a fertility unit on every proverbial corner, but when you look at the information closely you see enormous variables of scale and specialisation. A plethora of small units are handling perhaps only one or two treatments in contrast to some of the larger and better-known centres of excellence offering the full range of available treatment. But then such large centres are frequently overworked and overstretched.

This fragmentation of resources reflects a (designed) disintegration of the Health Service along with many other institutions of the welfare state. Divided and ruled, fertility professionals tend to ferret away each in his or her own corner, busy looking for strategies to boost their competitive edge. It would make far more sense if there were simply, for example, 10 large fertility centres in the UK which could attract all the country's medical expertise and funding. They could operate as reliable and respected environments where as patients we could feel like people wanting children rather than consumers in a booming market of 'luxury' medicine. Instead we have a system which is open to exploitation.

A Word of Caution about Clinical Success Rate Statistics

With clinics operating in a competitive environment, their own livelihood depends on the combined factor of an HFEA License and clients (patients). Clients naturally tend to gravitate towards businesses which are successful, and a fertility clinic's results are the slippery gauge by which people naturally make their decisions. If you are going to part with large sums of money (and even if not), you will quite understandably want to know what your odds are. You may then find your Consultant extremely unwilling to answer your questions conclusively. Why?

Statistical tables are a kind of mathematical nonsense. The HFEA publish painstaking statistical success rate charts each year, constantly trying to break down the information in ever more imaginative combinations. The truth is, it is extremely hard to achieve a statistical prognosis since there are so many factors to take into account in each individual case: age of partners, fertility problems, general health, to name but a few. Statistics only give a generalised picture, and when it comes to columns of figures, life just isn't like that – certainly not its creation! For example, a centre of excellence might boast a 20 per cent IVF success rate. But this clinic might have an upper age limit which is lower than that of other clinics the statistic compares to. Then you have to consider: what were the infertility causes of the patients quoted in the statistic? Were most of them straightforward (such as tubal damage only) and how many 'difficult' cases (such as low sperm plus endometriosis) does it include? Then again, cases of tubal damage tend to show the highest success rate, but if a woman is 40 years old with tubal damage her chances may be as low as 5–10 per cent. In short, published statistics can be really unhelpful and even misleading. They are also easy to massage.

The mixed economy of health care has also made it difficult to establish a consensus on an appropriate definition of success: should it be fertilisation, a clinical pregnancy (a positive pregnancy test), an established pregnancy, a live birth or a healthy baby? The answer depends on whose interest is being served.
NAOMI PFEFFER, *THE STORK AND THE SYRINGE* (POLITY PRESS, 1993)

When choosing a clinic (if you indeed have a choice), consider the experience of the unit first and foremost. Then look at the environment itself. You will be spending a lot of stressful time in it. Does it have the facilities you would expect? Do the staff seem overstretched or do they have time for you as an individual? Do you feel comfortable there? Is it convenient to get to (you will be having to go there in the early hours of the morning and in the middle of the night)? If you have a car, does the clinic provide convenient parking facilities? Is it independent from a maternity or gynaecological ward or may you have to suffer the torture of sitting in waiting rooms alongside bulging bellies or women seeking abortions? Is the unit vigilant about being a chemical-free environment, since chemicals such as deodorants and perfumes can affect the success of your treatment?

How Can You Get the Answer to the Simple Question 'What Are Our Chances?'

When you have decided on a clinic, use your first consultancy (once your infertility has been diagnosed) to compile a statistic that is specific to your individual profile as a couple.

Research is currently being conducted at the Hammersmith Hospital into seeing whether a computer model can be developed to give couples seeking IVF treatment an individual prognosis based on their specific infertility factors. This research is being devised from data from 9,000 IVF cycles stored on computer. Even so, the tailor-made success rate predicted will be subject to the many unknown factors involved which currently remain in the power of Nature herself.

So, until this research is completed and proven to work, I advise you to consider the published statistics for each clinic as only part of the picture you want to build in reaching an informed decision about whether to pursue treatment and where.

The User's Guide to UK Clinics (Appendix, *page 245*) includes just some of the questions you need to ask. If you are interested in the statistics (which I have deliberately excluded), contact the HFEA and ask for their Patient's Guide to UK Clinics (*see page 284*).

First Contact with a Clinic

This will be by phone. You will probably be in a sensitive and vulnerable mood when you call and need to be alerted to some of the frustrations that might immediately hit you:

1. The number listed for the clinic or unit might have changed from the one listed in the HFEA Guide or the one in this book.
2. The number might be the main hospital switchboard and the person answering may not understand your request. Ask to be put in touch with either 'the fertility clinic', the 'assisted conception unit', the 'IVF unit' or, if you are not sure, the obstetrics and gynaecology ward where someone will certainly know how to get you connected to the right person in the right place.
3. Be prepared to be told that there is a long waiting list for a first appointment with the Consultant.
4. Ask the administrator or co-ordinator to whom you are speaking whether they would answer some questions you may have about the clinic (*NB*: make a list beforehand).

Ask whether it might be possible to visit even before your first appointment, and be sure that the clinic sends you its brochure.

Questions to Ask a Clinic

Getting a picture of the clinic's ethos, experience and practice involves some research. There are certain kinds of information which provide clues to their general attitudes, sexual politics, financing. For instance, clinics involved in research may be at the cutting edge of new technology. You might want to know where money from their private patients is going (for example, is it direct to the Consultants or does it help to fund the clinic's perhaps under-funded public sector practice? Does private money go into research projects, for instance?) Ask the clinic to explain this. It is your right to know.

Discount packages: Be very careful to check what these actually mean. Packages may appear advantageous but might have hidden traps. For instance, a clinic may offer a discount package of four treatment cycles but wouldn't refund you any money if you became pregnant successfully after your first attempt. You need to consider your options carefully here.

Some questions are covered in the User's Guide (*pages 245–75*). Others you should ask might include:

- Are costs quoted inclusive (of drugs, blood tests, sperm tests and consultancy fees, professional counselling, etc.)?
- What tests would they conduct?
- What restrictions do they have?
- How many times would you have to visit during the course of tests and treatment?
- How does the clinic treat you as a couple?
- What is the clinic's live birth rate?
- Will the Consultant remain involved in your treatment throughout?
- Who are the clinic's donors of eggs and sperm?
- Does the clinic have an egg sharing scheme?
- Is the clinic involved in research and, if so, what?
- How large is the clinic's staff?
- How many patients does the clinic treat each year?
- Is the clinic sharing facilities with a maternity unit or gynaecological ward?
- What happens if you get pregnant – that is, is the clinic part of a hospital which would offer you antenatal care?
- Is there a patient's support group and, if so, how can you get in touch with them?

You might also wish to build up a more detailed understanding of some of the medical choices a clinic makes, for example use of drugs in treatments such as DI and IVF, why the clinic may favour one technique over another, whether they use a vaginal or abdominal ultrasound scanner, etc.

The Clinic as Temple

Sammy Lee, author of *Counselling in Male Infertility*, suggests that fertility clinics are modern-day temples, complete with their high-priests, laws and rituals.[VI] And you, the subfertile, will come to these places full of anxiety, hope and determination. There's no point telling you how you will cope, for obviously each individual and couple will respond to the whole process in different ways. What is important is that you come to your treatment as fully informed as possible and able to negotiate the experience so that you can feel you have retained your dignity and remained in control.

Choosing a Clinic

In reality only those couples who are paying for their treatment privately will have any fundamental choices about which clinic to opt for and why. There may be certain cases of NHS patients being able to use the Patient's Charter to their advantage, but you may well find that where you get treated will boil down to geography and Health Service economics. Those of you who are private patients are effectively consumers in the ART market and it is important that you consider some facts before rushing into any decisions. The clinical environment is obviously important for you to feel happy and comfortable in, and this includes not only its location and amenities but the human environment of its medical and secretarial staff.

Things to Expect at the IVF Clinic

Each IVF clinic will have its own ethos, atmosphere, staffing structure and procedures. Some will automatically build professional specialist counselling into your treatment, others will offer this as an extra (and charge for it). Some will give you information sessions in groups with other couples, some will only do this on an individual basis. Some will be based alongside a fertility clinic, some may be separate. Some may be situated uncomfortably close to an obstetrics and gynaecological clinic, meaning that whilst waiting for results or scans you may feel tormented by the sight of pregnant women or women with babies and small children. Many clinics will display photographs of babies they have 'produced' like awards of distinction. This may inspire you or depress you. It is obviously meant to do the former, but really it would be more honest to show the pictures of babies born successfully alongside portraits of the many unfortunate couples for whom treatment hasn't worked.

There are things you can do to gain a sense of control over the easily intimidating aspects of IVF. It does no harm to discuss any of the following with the clinic staff:

Sperm Samples

These are generally required to be given at the clinic at specified times. Some clinics can only offer a toilet for this, whereas the richer ones may have special rooms. Sometimes these rooms are fitted out with pornography – magazines and videos – and seem more like a hotel room than a hospital. The porn is there to help men who mightn't otherwise be able to ejaculate on cue. It is the subject of quiet controversy in the infertile community and you should consider how you feel about this. If you have strong feelings, religious or ethical objections about the use of pornography in the making of your baby, you can as a couple do the following:

- Request that the man's partner be present at all sperm sample-givings.
- Request a spermicide-free condom and take the sperm sample as the result of love-making at home. Normally this is only permitted a) when there are cultural or religious objections to masturbation b) if you live near enough to the hospital to get the sperm to the lab quickly. You may be asked to pay extra for the special condoms.

The problem for me is that solo-sex is rather meaningless ... It leads easily to a sense of silliness, anti-climax or even loss of dignity, and hence – more practically – loss of erection ... The fact that the hospital has deliberately provided sexy magazines, independently of any moral counter-pressures, signals that King's people understand what the problem is for donors, on a human scale. The message, intentionally or otherwise is: 'We know it might be harder to produce your sample than you thought; we can't exactly come in there and help, so here's some substitute encouragement.'
SPERM DONOR, KING'S COLLEGE HOSPITAL, LONDON

Injections

You will be offered the option of administering these yourself, following clear guidelines from your clinic. For those who would prefer medical supervision, consult with your clinic and your GP about the most practical way of organising this as your GP may be prepared to adminster.

Making Embryo Transfer Special

Embryo transfer, the moment you will feel you begin to 'carry' your potential baby, is an extremely sensitive and even beautiful occasion (despite the bright lights, technology, the fact that you will be surrounded by people wearing surgical gowns and J-cloths on their heads and that it's all over in a flash). One thing you must ask for is to look at your embryos on the screen before they are inserted. Also, ask for a scan photograph, which you will probably treasure. You may also request beforehand to have music playing and bring in the tape of your choice. Not only will this help to add a human and spiritual touch to highly medicalised proceedings, but it will help you to feel familiar and relaxed.

In November 2000 the British media became obsessed with the Thompsons' case, a couple who successfully sued their IVF clinic for transferring 3 embryos resulting in the birth of healthy triplets. Columnists, family values campaigners and medical experts vented spleen on the Thompsons, claiming variously that they were greedy, uncaring parents and ungrateful for their 'blessings'. The attack, unsurprisingly, demonised Mrs Thompson in particular. She, meanwhile, has argued that her claim was 'not about money. It was about choice, and having my choice respected' (*Daily Telegraph* 18th November 2000). The point was that she had requested a maximum of 2 embryos to be transferred and has been under sedation when she 'consented' to 3. Juliet Tizzard of Progress has argued cogently in support of Mrs Thompson's position. 'If a contraceptive is faulty and a conception follows, it seems fair that the manufacturer of the contraceptive take responsibility. This case is no different in this respect ... in other areas of medicine patient choice is championed. Why can't it be the same for reproductive medicine?'
BIONEWS, 20TH NOVEMBER 2000

Consent Forms

You will be asked to sign consent forms before treatment. These are vital documents since they relate to your wishes about the future use of your eggs, sperm and embryos in donation and research. You do of course have the option to allow your gametes and embryos to perish without further intervention. You may also wish to offer them for donation, though this offer may be declined if you exceed the upper age limits. Instead of grappling with understanding them at the eleventh hour (as you are about to undergo treatment), ask the clinic if they might provide you with samples of consent forms beforehand. Read them well. Ask the counsellor or co-ordinator to explain anything you don't understand.

1. As at September 1996.
2. Only 1 baby born by this method in the UK (in 1995). Current HFEA moratorium on further attempts.
3. Some women have opted to conduct their own insemination with a known donor, quite independently from the medical establishment, and have succeeded in getting pregnant. Many lesbian couples have achieved families this way. The risk of the AIDS virus has tended to medicalise the process more, as women seek assurance that the sperm they are using isn't infected with HIV.
4. PZD no longer has a role in contemporary management of IVF.
5. Private surrogacy arrangements must be as old as history, particularly between family members. This quote from the Bible is part of the story of the sisters Rachel and Leah. Jacob loved Rachel but, as a result of a complex marital arrangement with her father Laban, was made to marry Leah first. Jacob had seven children by Leah. He also had two by Leah's maid and two by Rachel's maid Bilbah, children both Leah and Rachel mothered as their own. Rachel was barren, but finally God answered her prayer for a baby of her own and she bore Jacob a son, Joseph.

CHAPTER (3)

Feelings

Cuckoo Calling

If she could feel, spring would appal
the world running its egg-and-sperm race
the birdcall blatant with demand.

She is stone: black; heavy; inert.
Where flesh was, moss grows.
Where hope was there is a gap.

In the gap the cuckoo came calling
a flap of wing among trees
and fast and unseen filled it.

JACQUELINE BROWN, *THINKING EGG* (LITTLEWOOD ARC, 1993)

(1) Infertility and the Couple

The point about babies and children is that all of us have a relationship of some kind with the *idea* of them. Whether we desire them or not, from quite an early age we will have thought about whether we see ourselves as parents in the future. Regardless of gender, race or sexuality, our adult identity will then be profoundly bound up with whether or not we breed.

Most, though not all, infertility treatment is undergone within a heterosexual relationship. Whether or not this relationship has followed the conventional path of marriage, the majority of men and women who establish an intimate and committed unit do so with the shared desire to create a family. There are of course the important and not-to-be-forgotten minority: Those couples who actually opt for a child-free life together (often faced with adjusting people's expectations of them to breed and an assumption of pity that they are childless). Then there are gay couples for whom the choice to have a baby of their own is fraught with medical, legislative and social obstacles. There are those couples stressed by the fact that one but not both crave a child. If their relationship survives it can only be through compromise. Lastly there are single women who for reasons of choice or accident don't have a partner with whom to breed, as the biological clock pounds cruelly loud in their ears. They face a difficult choice to try and conceive without a life partner and, if successful, with the rigours and demands of single-parenting.

Each case brings its own pains and challenges. I am dealing in this chapter primarily with the heterosexual involuntarily childless as the largest single group who seek Assisted Conception via Licensed Clinics (for lesbian and single-parenting please refer to *pages 238–9 and 239*, and to access sympathetic counsellors see, for example, the Women's Therapy Centre in the Useful Addresses, page 280).

Infertility is an emotional minefield, and either partner within a couple may ignite at any moment. Failing to conceive a baby is devastating. For the woman, each month will be an agony of hoping, waiting and grief. This is particularly so for the older woman:

She will begin to count off her life in months, or, more precisely, in ovulations. Ovulations come, on average, every 28 days. So, while the rest of the world works to the universally recognised calendar of days, weeks, months, years, all that ends for the older woman who hopes for a child ... most critically, she has a sense of being hermetically sealed in this private timeframe. The cycles have a beginning and ending that, for her and her only, resonate with a giant thud through her body.
PAMELA ARMSTRONG, *BEATING THE BIOLOGICAL CLOCK – THE JOYS AND CHALLENGES OF LATE MOTHERHOOD* (HEADLINE, 1996)

But feelings of crashing disappointment associated with monthly periods will be common to women of any age trying and failing to make a baby naturally.

For the man, the emotional process at this stage will probably be quite different. Most men assume that fertility problems are the woman's. This is a myth. Recent statistics show that male fertility problems constitute 32 per cent of single causes of infertility, whilst 20–25 per cent of couples have a combined factor problem, meaning that in total 50 per cent of infertile couple's problems may involve a male problem.

The diagnosis of male subfertility is a big blow to a person's self esteem. In some, even in cases of azoospermia, there is complete denial. Often they will ask 'why me?' It is almost as if the answer to this question will in some way salve the pain ... Inevitably there are also issues over the apportionment of blame. It is common for the female partner to express relief and a shifting of burden when the spotlight falls on the male partner. There exists also the issues of 'is God punishing me?' and 'what have I done to deserve this?' A common summation of all these feelings, especially within the medical setting, is a growing feeling of total uselessness. There seems so little that can be done for male infertility. Any treatment options seem to centre entirely on the blameless partner (the female). This results in the man feeling marginalised.

*When looking at cultural differences, there is an added emotional charge,
for example Middle Eastern men often cannot accept that they are the cause
of infertility.*
SAMMY LEE, *COUNSELLING IN MALE INFERTILITY* (BLACKWELL SCIENCE, 1996)

The poet Benjamin Zephaniah discovered in 1992 that he was chronically
infertile due to the complete absence of sperm in his semen. His 'coming
out' as a (black) infertile man was a brave act since there is commonly so
much machismo attached to the idea of male potency, a persistent
confusion between fertility and virility, and the traditional male's dynastic
urge to reproduce. He was the subject of a TV documentary *Shooting Blanks*
about male infertility and has written movingly of his feelings about
childlessness:

*I have devised my own self-help plan – surrounding myself with animals,
keeping busy, and enjoying sex. Being unable to become the father that I would
like does not make me feel an incomplete man but it makes me feel an
incomplete human being.*

*I reject the idea that my wanting is about machismo ... I want to be a
daddy; it's the greatest ambition I've ever had and it haunts me every day.*

*On bad days I look into the heavens and wonder why Nazis and child
molesters can have children but I can't.*
THE OBSERVER, 22ND JANUARY 1994

Zephaniah is an exceptional man because he has not only admitted his
condition but done so publicly, even trying to raise consciousness in the
black male community about infertility in general and the desperate
shortage of black sperm donors. The majority of men can find the news that
they have a low, poor or absent sperm count devastating to their pride and
manhood and may respond with disbelief and denial from which they may
find it very hard to shift.

Childless

Strong biceps
Firm thighs
Big bottom
Sexy eyes,
Fast

On the track
Strong like
A lion
Good Kung-Fu feet
And healthy hair.
Strong triceps
No lie,
Rhymster
Nice guy,
A good healthy back
Great levels of iron,
There must be a baby
In there,
Somewhere,
There must be
A baby
In here.

BENJAMIN ZEPHANIAH, *PROPA PROPAGANDA* (BLOODAXE BOOKS, 1996)

Male pride or fertility factor aside, however, the fact is that the principal ordeal of Assisted Conception falls on the woman. With ART women's bodies remain the sites for medical intervention. It is her body that will be prodded, scanned, probed, injected, cut and invaded, and it will be her body coping with the effects of hormone treatment, anaesthetic and post-operative distress. This is not to belittle men's feelings but to remind us that whereas a man may be going through intense trauma, his distress (unless he is taking hormone drugs) will be psychological, emotional and empathetic. For a woman it is all this and more. In the case of low sperm count, a technique such as ICSI is actually giving fertile women the option to undergo the intervention of full IVF, drugs, surgery *et al.*, whilst the man need only produce a sperm sample. The combination of Nature and Technology conspires to make the woman physiologically suffer subfertility more directly than the man, and this in turn can have a huge impact on the couple. Whilst the man might feel rage at his loss of manhood, parenthood and the spectre of his genetic death, the woman may feel the added rage that she has to put her body through such hurdles. Her rage might be compounded by feelings of anger at the injustice of male privilege and power and the fact that she is more than likely to be receiving treatment by male consultants and doctors.

In cases where the woman has the fertility dysfunction, she may feel a real fear that the man will leave her if she doesn't produce a child. There are some cultures in which a childless woman is simply traded in for a newer model. Even in more liberal Western communities, women's roles and identities are still intricately bound up with bearing children. Biological drive and the biological clock can eventually catch up with even the most determinedly independent woman in her late thirties. Men can afford to be circumspect. They have time on their side and choice with which to play the field.

Some Areas of Especial Difficulty for the Couple

Throughout infertility investigations and treatment, couples may hit flashpoints of stress and difficulty where things seem to just blow up and rows happen. These may be when dealing with:

Sperm Samples

One area of treatment where men can feel vulnerable and humiliated is in giving sperm samples. In some units this procedure will be extremely clinical and take place in a toilet. In others he may find himself in a furnished room kitted out with pornography. Whilst this is provided to help men to masturbate on cue in the sterile and unsexy environment of the hospital, there is something really tacky about the idea that, with ART, babies may be being conceived in response to hard-core. Some women and men get very angry at this, and some men cannot even bring themselves to tell their partners about 'the room'.

Scheduled Sex

When trying to conceive naturally (guided or not by a doctor) according to charts and calendars, sex can be extremely hard to broach and even harder to enjoy. Many men find the pressure makes them temporarily impotent, whilst many women are so upset at their partners' avoidance or ignorance of 'the time of the month' that rows erupt before they even get as far as sexual contact. Scheduled sex is particularly difficult when you are planning a Post-Coital Test since the timing needs to be so precise (*see pages 25–6*).

Hormone Treatment

Many women undergoing hormone treatment experience a (temporary) emotional upheaval. Their whole system is being intentionally retuned and the result can be volcanic: huge mood swings and a feeling of being in the grip of forces beyond your control. It has been described by some women as 'PMT times 10'.

Donor Gametes

One of the most emotionally sensitive issues of all for a couple to negotiate is that of donor gametes. Either partner may have very strong feelings about this, but research suggests that it is particularly hard for men to come to terms with another man's sperm going inside the woman's body to make a baby, whilst women seem to accept more easily the idea of social rather than genetic mothering.

Surrogacy

This is perhaps the hardest option to take in wanting a child who is at least half genetically yours (*NB*: surrogacy can also be used with IVF to gestate a child that is the genetic child of both parents). Surrogacy is likely to raise all kinds of difficult feelings, including jealousy (female partner to surrogate and vice-versa) and anxiety (the law states that the surrogate mother is the legal mother, so she has the right to change her mind once pregnancy has been achieved).

Waiting

The hardest thing for both of you to experience singly and together is all the waiting involved:

> for an appointment for tests
> for tests
> for the results of tests
> for referrals
> for more tests
> for the results of these tests
> for more tests
> for the results of these tests
> for an operation
> for the result of the operation
> for a funding decision
> for getting started on treatment
> for tests
> for egg collection
> for results
> for embryo transfer
> for pregnancy
> for the pregnancy to be viable/or not
> for the pregnancy to be safe/or not
> for a baby to be born/or not
> for more tests?
> (take it again, from the top?)

Working Things Out Together

The best thing you can do as a couple is to *communicate*. If either of you bottles things up it will only come out in the end, probably in a more chaotic and destructive way. Don't be afraid of fighting, but make sure you try to resolve your disagreements. Men are advised to stand by and take some deep breaths. A woman going through fertility treatment is likely to be emotionally unrecognisable at times. You both need support, but she will need especial understanding and forbearance. She is going through both a physical and psychological upheaval. Try and find ways to counter stress together. Go for long walks and use these to discuss your feelings with each other. Plan special holidays or breaks together during treatment (provided doctors advise it). Be good to yourselves and each other. Try and make the treatment time a special time. Don't lose touch with each other whatever friction there may be. Use friends, family, patients' support groups and/or a counsellor to help you both get through the low times. The most important thing is not to repress any of your fears, angers or anxieties but to look at everything head on. There may be a time when you both need to re-evaluate your desire for a baby in the light of the experience of diagnosis/prognosis/failed treatment cycle(s). Don't be afraid of saying anything. It's always better to speak these things sooner rather than later. Remember ART is not a factory nor a treadmill. It is stoppable at any point of exhaustion, when you feel you can no longer cope, or when you know your relationship needs a break.

Times of acute stress during an infertility crisis might be:
Whilst undergoing investigations
Whilst waiting to see a Consultant
Whilst waiting for exploratory operations
Whilst waiting for any result
Whilst taking hormones
Whilst waiting for fertilisation results
Whilst waiting for pregnancy results
Whilst getting bad news

Assisted Conception: A Coping Budget

When weighing up whether or not to proceed with some of the more invasive fertility treatments such as IVF and IUI with donor gametes, try budgeting the real cost to you and your partner. You could give each item marks out of 10, or just jot some notes down next to them. Do this together. Add your own items. You could then devise another for your alternatives. Writing things down can make things clearer and help you talk as a couple about hidden feelings, fears and anxieties. Eg:

The Real Cost to Me/Us:
money
time
stress
pressure
anxiety
energy
health
relationship

It is really worth putting in the time to work things out together before, not during or after treatment, so as to avoid misunderstanding and conflict during a treatment cycle, when you will be feeling most vulnerable and possibly hormonally upset.

If you decide to go ahead with treatment you might want to decide together how many attempts you will go for. This will help you to feel more in control. Prepare yourselves to cope with each result in the context of your overall plan.

If you don't know at first how many times you will try, remember that many, many people don't make a baby on the first attempt and that the first attempt is often a diagnostic one for doctors and you to see how your body responds to each aspect of the treatment.

It is vital to know when to stop trying. Remember, you have choice. Don't be afraid of quitting at any stage. You aren't letting anyone down. It is *your* body and *your* life.

⑪ Coping: Counselling

Most people at some point in their lives have ideas of a dream child. Children when thinking of playing at mummy or daddy have an idea about a dream child. Most of us grow up with ideas of dream children at some point and then usually those who want a child have it and the dream child gets fed into reality and slowly the dream takes on a reality. But for people who can't have children there's never a resolution of the dream so is it any wonder how distressing it is? It is that process that really needs addressing, not just the mechanics but the symbolic.

SUE EMMY JENNINGS – DRAMATHERAPIST AND INFERTILITY COUNSELLOR

Infertility is a kind of death. However, unlike death, which whilst deeply painful to confront is part of a natural process, not being able to procreate when you want to feels cruelly unnatural. It is as if Nature has cheated us out of our birthright and we don't know how to cope with the rush of emotions that plague us.

Some of these intensely painful feelings may be of 'abnormality', 'difference' and, worst of all, 'failure'. Your body is letting you down, not performing and not producing as it should. The world is suddenly chock-full of mothers, of prams cocooning the excruciating beauty of babies, of playgrounds echoing with the laughter of children at play. All your friends are doing it or have done it. They seem to belong to a secret society of childcare schedules, maternal moans and parental pride. Even egg-stained and exhausted, you envy them to distraction as they clatter about their busy child-full lives as bona fide members of the human race. Meanwhile, you writhe inside in agony and despair at the great chasm in your own life. The impact of infertility hits us to the very core of our beings. A range of thoughts and pains may obsess us in response:

- We may grieve our genetic death, the fact that our genes will not continue.
- We may feel the essence of us – our sexuality – is suddenly arid, disabled, redundant.
- We may feel our 'insides' are derelict.
- We may feel that our creativity, so deeply connected to our sexuality, has ceased.
- We may feel that we are prevented from growing up ourselves by not having the experience of parenting.
- We may mourn the loss of our fertile identity that we have perhaps had since early childhood.
- We may suffer the loss of social identity and feel deviant, abnormal and subhuman for our difference.
- We may feel rage at our partner for their infertility or for what we imagine to be our infertility in their eyes.
- We may feel guilt for our previous lifestyle or the choices we have made, such as to postpone having children till our career was established.
- We may feel powerless and thwarted that our future is now blocked.

Things which may stimulate your pain:
Parks
Playgrounds
Schools
Families
Babygoods shops
Maternity wear shops
Doctors' waiting rooms
TV programmes, films, books, plays which include: children (happy or suffering) and/or families (especially happy ones)
any public places where people gather
pregnant women
births
deaths

You are neither mad to be feeling the welter of emotions that may arise, nor is it a sign of weakness, instability or incompetence to need counselling at some point during the course of your diagnosis, treatment and/or decision-making. Some of the most capable and successful people have been known to feel like emotional wrecks as a result of their subfertility. The stress on both the individual and the couple can be quite overwhelming. Experts acknowledge that the experience of fertility treatment either makes or breaks a couple. This is not necessarily because of some fundamental flaw in you or the relationship, but because infertility triggers so many other emotions, hurts our self-esteem, and alienates us from the majority of people's lives around us. In some cases the infertility problem may exacerbate an existing problem between you. In others the stress may be so extreme that a previously happy relationship simply cracks under the strain. On the other hand, a relationship can be significantly strengthened by having shared the infertility journey. It will prove to be a time in your lives where you may feel very raw and naked but where the very fact that you both have to expose your deepest selves, your sexuality, your reproductive systems, your dreams, your futures may create tremendous frankness, bonding and team-work. One of the few privileges of fertility treatment is the heightened state of awareness it forces us to bring to a process the majority of people take for granted or stumble upon in a state of unplanned semi-ignorance.

Infertile couples are dealing on a daily basis not so much with a medical condition that they have but more its consequences – that is, what they do not have – the lack of a child, children or control on forming the family they want. An outcome of their mutual love and affection. When you don't have something you really want generally people are upset, silenced, often angry or feel ignored and deprived, particularly when it is something that most people have without problem.

TIFFANY BLACK, ACU PATIENTS SUPPORT GROUP, KING'S COLLEGE HOSPITAL, LONDON

Things you may feel about your subfertility:
shock
disbelief
anger
powerlessness
regret
guilt
shame
anxiety
panic
frustration
bitterness
worthlessness
emptiness
confusion
despair
humiliation
jealousy
rage
vulnerability
a feeling of being:
    a failure
    overwhelmed
    lost
    blocked
    asexual/sexless
    incomplete
    robbed
    denied
    less than human
    suicidal

Infertility as Bereavement

Fairly recent studies on the effects of infant mortality alerted helping professionals to recognise patterns of grief. The need for the bereaved to go through stages of mourning and a process of ritual is a necessary part of healing. Without such expression, feelings remain unresolved and potentially destructive to the bereaved parent's life. This model has now been applied to infertility counselling. The unborn, lost, or dream baby is mourned and along with it the loss of parenthood that never was. Sue Emmy Jennings reckons this process of bereavement takes a lot of time. After all, we are never 'cured' of our infertility. Even if we eventually succeed in making a baby through the available technology, our bodies remain infertile and we may have experienced many losses along the way. We may have lost one of a twin or triplets *in utero*. We may have achieved a pregnancy and miscarried. We may have frozen embryos which we can't for some reason use. We may simply never have any hope of a baby at all.

Grieving is as natural as eating, drinking and breathing. It is a deeply-rooted instinct not only common to humans. We now know that some animals have their own bereavement rituals: whales keen, elephants have their graveyards and David Attenborough recently showed an extraordinary film of hippos mourning their dead at night. Dr Simon Fishel, Director of CARE told the audience at the 'Angels and Mechanics' Conference in June 1996 how a childless couple in their seventies came to him and said they wanted to leave their entire estate to the fertility clinic after their death. Still devastated by their childlessness, this was their way of 'letting go and moving on', of participating in the future and of saying goodbye.

You aren't being indulgent if you need to create a farewell ritual for your lost or unborn child(ren). Talk about it with your partner. Find something that has meaning for you both and don't be embarrassed to do it. It might be as simple as planting something in memory. You might find writing really helpful. You might write a letter to your unborn child and tell him/her how you feel. You might want to create an 'album' of memories – scans, hospital letters, etc., to keep. You may never look at it but at least you have marked something, reclaimed the emotional, spiritual and intensely personal reality of your 'ghost' babies and your own personal infertility experience.

We decided that we didn't want to use our frozen embryos because of the lack of medical evidence about the use of them in the long term. For months until we had access to them it was as though eight umbilical cords were flapping in the wind. I was in a state of real pain, loss and anger about them. I then realised they represented my only chance of having any more children. We decided to bury them in the garden and plant something special over them. I was touched and surprised that the embryologist at the hospital let me sit in a quiet room and have a little cry on receiving them. She told me that it was happening more and more, people retrieving their embryos to do something personal with them. It made me feel less mad and neurotic.
MOTHER OF AN IVF BABY

The Bereavement Model: Stages in Grieving
- shock, numbness, disbelief
- denial
- guilt, anger, hostility
- searching (for object of loss)
- facing reality.

The important thing to understand about this model is that it isn't a neat, linear journey from one phase to the next. People feel different things at different times and may move backwards and forwards through the different stages. For example, many men can't work right through the bereavement because they get stuck at a stage of denial from which they can't move on. The overall aim is to experience facing reality even if the idea of neatly drawing a line under it can never really be achieved. The point is to be enabled to find a way of continuing your life, with the loss of your dream baby or babies integrated into your memory as part of the many profound experiences which go to make you what you are.

People won't necessarily understand your bereavement, particularly if you have secondary infertility or if you have created a family through adoption, fostering or surrogacy. Ignore their ignorance. Protect yourself from their trivialising of your deepest feelings. Concentrate quietly and privately on what you need to do and say to help you come to terms with your sense of loss. Enlist the support of trusted family and friends if it feels right. Otherwise do it with your partner or on your own if your partner doesn't feel the same as you.

I knew a woman who decided if she couldn't have babies she'd grow a garden. She started the garden while she was still seeing me and she was bringing in

little plans of borders and things. It was so creative. Every now and then I get a postcard saying 'by the way, so and so's grown!'
SUE EMMY JENNINGS

Striving for a Second Child

You may find people simply can't understand a) your stress and pain at failing to conceive a second child or, in their ignorance b) why you aren't producing a second child since this is such a 'norm' in our culture. You may also find the fact that you are already a parent provokes jealousy rather than solidarity with fellow infertiles who (in their own despair at being totally childless) may not comprehend what's going on for you at all.

People would constantly try and get to grips with their grief for me by saying 'you have a child'. And I would just say to people 'look, I just want to regurgitate on you. Just be there, just listen to me, that's all I want. I want another child. I have this beautiful daughter but I want this child so badly.' I would say to mum 'can't you understand the pressure we are going through?' and she'd just belittle it and that just hurt so much.
WOMAN UNDERGOING ICSI

Significant Occasions which may be very hard for you:
  Religious holidays, such as:
    Christmas
    Ramadan
    Pesach
    Diwali
    etc.
  Weddings
  Confirmations
  Circumcisions
  Christenings or newborn ceremonies
  Barmitzvas and Batmitzvas
  Births (friends', relatives')
  Holidays abroad
  Birthdays (your own, children's)
  Anniversaries (of, for example, abortions, the loss of a baby or child, miscarriage, a failed IVF attempt)

What Is Counselling?

People need to be aware that they don't have to be problem-driven to use the counselling service.
JENNIFER HUNT, SENIOR COUNSELLOR, HAMMERSMITH HOSPITAL

Counselling is different from psychotherapy or psychoanalysis. The latter both assume deep disturbances rooted in childhood and sexuality, requiring long-term and in-depth accessing of repressed memory and emotion as a key to healing. Counselling starts from the idea of addressing the immediate issue in people's lives (such as infertility) and exploring any inhibiting, destructive or painful feelings associated with it. During a relatively short course of sessions (agreed in advance), the counsellor offers an opportunity to air, discuss, problem-solve and generally find a way of coping with 'matters arising'. There are of course areas of overlap between counselling and therapy. But let's for now take 'professional counselling' to mean the basic dictionary definition of the word 'counsel': *advice, consultation, assistance* and *guidance.*

Why the Need for a Counsellor as Well as a Doctor?

Infertility is a life-crisis and, to the newcomer, the field of ART can be baffling, alarming, traumatising and alienating. It tends to provoke many issues of an emotional, moral, spiritual and ethical nature for the patient. For example, a busy Consultant treating scores of patients each week may discuss donor gametes with you in a seemingly casual and detached way because these techniques are the daily tools of his or her trade. And, as we well know, doctors aren't always sensitive to emotions. They also have power over you. You may feel very confused, disturbed and anxious. You may feel that if you don't go along with his or her advice you will never have a child of your own. And you may feel that if you don't show avid keenness you will not be considered serious candidates for treatment.

What you will need is time and space to take stock of any news that has hit you, to understand fully the medical issues and options, and to reach an informed decision with your partner about how to proceed. You aren't expected, nor should you ever be advised, to make such decisions on the spot during the course of a medical consultation.

Counselling provides a quiet space where you can mull over those things that are worrying you and get the support and information you need to proceed to a decision with which you feel comfortable.

What Does a Counselling Session Involve?

The counsellor can see you individually or as a couple. You may wish to request specifically that your counsellor be a man or a woman. Where a mixed-gender team is available this shouldn't be a problem. There's no 'right way' or 'wrong way' to use counselling. The counsellor should be taking cues from you. He or she should refrain from directing you, and work with whatever feelings or problems you bring to the session. It is worth bearing in mind that, as with all professions, there are many different styles and methods of professional counselling. Some counsellors work with a simple talking-out method, whereas some might use other resources – drawing, chart-making, role-play, etc. – to help you sort out your feelings. The important thing is that you feel comfortable with your counsellor and helped by your sessions.

Seeing a Counsellor Doesn't Mean There's Anything 'Wrong' with You

As we have seen, there is a danger that infertility treatment over-medicalises the natural process of reproduction. Counselling in turn certainly shouldn't imply any pathologising of your infertility as a mental condition. There is no such thing as 'an infertile type of person'. Infertility is not a mental problem, neither a neurosis nor a psychosis. The fact is that you or/and your partner are having problems with the functioning of part or parts of your body. This dysfunction may be causing you a range of very turbulent emotions and you may need to talk these feelings through with someone trained to understand all aspects of what you are undergoing.

Infertility Counselling and the HFEA

The HF & E Act states that all people receiving licensed treatment must, before consenting to treatment, be given 'a suitable opportunity to receive proper counselling about the implications of taking the proposed steps''. The HFEA Code of Practice elaborates on this, by first setting out that counselling should be clearly distinguished from the giving of information (which should be given to everyone), the normal giving of advice by a clinician to a person seeking treatment, and the process of assessing people's eligibility for being a client or donor. The three types of counselling it recommends are:

a. *implications counselling*: this aims to enable the people concerned to understand the implications of the proposed course of action for themselves, for their family, and for any children born as a result;
b. *support counselling*: this aims to give emotional support at times of particular stress, such as when there is a failure to achieve pregnancy;
c. *therapeutic counselling*: this aims to help people to cope with the consequences of infertility and treatment, and to help them to resolve the problems which these may cause. It includes helping people to adjust their expectations and to accept their situation.

Centres **must** make implications counselling available to everyone.''

The fact is that infertility counselling is a new and emerging specialisation and that the HFEA guidelines, the practice of counsellors themselves and their status in the profession remains sources of debate within the profession.

We cannot get away from the medical hierarchy which is still male dominated. So you have a male dominated medical profession and a female dominated counselling profession really struggling to communicate with each other ... the counsellor has never been defined ... they're often seen by the doctor as the tea and sympathy person. What I call the 'would-you-just', you know: 'Mrs Smith is feeling very upset, would you just have a chat.'
SUE EMMY JENNINGS

Some Things Worth Knowing about Counsellors in the Fertility Clinic Setting

The status of counsellors in a clinical team might be low despite efforts on the part of the counselling profession. Some high-flying doctors, particularly those who are completely engrossed in the technological advances of Assisted Reproduction, may not value the counselling process enough. Clinics might be too money-orientated, making people pay too much for counselling. Also they may be interpreting the HFEA guidelines to mean different things, so it is worth considering some of the following issues which may concern you.

What Is the Counsellor's Role?

As regards 'Information', many counsellors say that they consider one of their jobs to be that of explaining medical information which has been given to the patient(s) by the doctor. The doctor may have given expert advice (counsel), but unless that advice is fully comprehended then it isn't advice but undigestible and potentially overwhelming information. So it isn't only doctors who can work at the information-end of a patient's treatment process. I know of at least one hospital where it is the Co-ordinator, essentially an administrator, who frequently finds herself answering patients' need for demystification and explanation. Because she is always there as the patients' first port-of-call, they trust her and will ask her things which she is perfectly capable of explaining. Technically it is not the Professional Counsellor's job to give advice as such, for example to say, 'If I were you I would go for IVF treatment.' However, professional Fertility Counsellors are medically informed and would certainly consider one of their functions to be to enable you to reach a position of informed choice.

Counselling and Patient Assessment

One area of greatest controversy is the counsellor's role in (Social) Assessment. For those counsellors working under the British Association for Counselling's Code of Practice, a confidentiality clause exists which means that assessment simply can't be part of their work. However, other counsellors may be involved in the Assessment process. A good and ethical counsellor should make it clear to you from the start that there may be an assessment process going on, and what the bounds of confidentiality are in the counselling context. You as the patient can then choose what to talk about. Some clinics will refer the patient for an assessment outside the clinic, as in cases of previous psychiatric illness. So it is vital that you are aware of your counsellor's role in your treatment plans. Don't be frightened off by this. Remember, you are in control.

There is no question of empowering the client in the counsellor-client relationship: the client is already empowered. If there is no empowerment there can be no counselling.

ROBERT SILMAN, 'WHAT IS INFERTILITY COUNSELLING?', *INFERTILITY COUNSELLING* (ED. SUE EMMY JENNINGS; BLACKWELL SCIENCE, 1995)

At What Point in Your Treatment Should a Counsellor Be Consulted?

In an ideal world many counsellors would like to be properly valued within the clinic's team and be there for the patient at the very start of any investigations or diagnosis. They feel this would remove the sting and normalise the role of counselling as part of the overall treatment. But in larger and busier clinics this is rarely the case for reasons of time, money and logistics, but you may be lucky to find a clinic that can offer you this service. Another reason it is good to see a counsellor early on is that it is very often precisely during the course of all the tests and operations which you may have to go through to reach a diagnosis that you will be feeling most frightened, stressed and confused. Your needs at this stage will be slightly different than when you are at a point of being diagnosed and offered options which you need to absorb and consider.

You wish there was a kind of kit you could be given for knowing how to cope and what to expect.

MAN WHOSE PARTNER WAS BOOKED FOR A LAPAROSCOPY AS PART OF FERTILITY TESTS

Is Counselling Free?

The only way for counselling to be truly accessible to everyone is for it to be built into the cost of overall treatment. Some clinics do offer a free service, whilst others don't. Some may have found loopholes in the HFEA Code of Practice so that the person designated to deliver Implications Counselling may not be a trained counsellor. You are well advised to ask right at the beginning of your relationship with a clinic what their counselling service consists of and, if it is an added cost, how much it will be. If there is a charge you may prefer to see your GP and find out if his or her practice has an in-house counsellor whom you would be eligible to see. Or you may choose to find your own counsellor outside of the clinic.

Therapeutic Counselling

Therapeutic Counselling is about dealing with your deepest feelings provoked by subfertility, treatment (or not) and success in having a baby (or not). The HFEA Code of Practice guidelines are unclear as to who should be offering Therapeutic Counselling, and suggest that in 'appropriate cases' patients should be referred for specialist counselling outside of the treatment centre. The current lack of training in Infertility Counselling means that where the clinic can provide specialists they will be coming from a wide range of backgrounds and training. Ask about this. You may have strong feelings or views about the method of Therapeutic Counselling you want to work with, and the clinic may be able to offer you a choice.

If the stress of your situation has created or exacerbated profound problems in your relationship you may wish to seek other therapeutic choices. RELATE (*see page 280*), whilst not working with infertility per se, are experts at working with couples. If you belong to a certain faith, you should find out whether there is a counselling service or relationship-guidance service within your religious organisation. You can also contact ISSUE or CHILD (*see page 279*), who offer counselling support and networks.

The Future of Infertility Counselling

Infertility counsellors may be nurses, social workers, clerics or trained psychotherapists and counsellors in other areas. Until very recently there was no formal training in Infertility Counselling. However, BICA (British Infertility Counselling Association) and BFS (British Fertility Society) have now jointly started a training and Accreditation Programme for Infertility Counsellors, which they hope will lead to some uniform standards.

If You Don't Want to See a Counsellor

There may be reasons why you don't want to take advantage of the clinic's counselling service. You may have your own ways of coping, you may have your own therapist, you may have family and friends who give you all the support you need. You may have a whole range of personal resources, creative and otherwise, which you know how to utilise. That's fine, but I do recommend that you go at least once to see the clinic's counsellor just to check out whether or not you might find it of special benefit.

(III) Coping: Networks and Patient Support Groups

National Organisations and Helplines

Whether undergoing investigation, contemplating treatment, grieving, considering adoption – indeed at whatever stage, it is worth thinking about using the various support systems that exist both locally and nationally. If you don't feel like being part of a group and going to meetings, you may find the services of charities such as ISSUE and CHILD really useful. Not only will they put you in touch with laypeople who have experienced what you are going through, but they offer professional advice and information. There are also numerous Helplines (*see pages 276–85*) for people who are needing advice and support on particular issues and experiences. These are often run from people's own homes, so don't (unless a 24-hour open line is stated) call in the middle of the night. If you do feel desperate or suicidal at unsocial hours, The Samaritans can be helpful for just 'offloading' your pain and stress until you can speak to an appropriate person (counsellor, friend, helpline, contact). Helplines have invariably been set up by people who have first-hand experience and they will really understand your distress, confusion or need for advice.

The two major national organisations to support people with infertility problems are:

ISSUE (The National Fertility Association)

A registered charity founded 20 years ago by a couple with infertility problems. ISSUE provides an individually-tailored and confidential service to people at whatever stage in their infertility crisis they might be. For a registration fee of £30 (at time of writing) benefits include:

- *Information:* independent, relevant information on all aspects of infertility and related topics. This is provided through a range of over 30 factsheets in addition to other articles. A regular magazine contains readers' stories, topical news items and medical articles.
- *Coping strategies:* providing help in the way of contacts, a network of helpful members, and counsellors.
- *Support Line:* a telephone counselling service where you are put in touch with qualified and experienced counsellors whom you can consult on medical, legal, psychological or relationship problems.
- *Adoption and inter-country adoption:* although not an adoption agency, ISSUE puts its members in touch with adoption experts and others who have successfully adopted, as well as keeping abreast of adoption issues worldwide.
- *Public and professional awareness:* ISSUE raises professional awareness and creates public understanding of infertility difficulties by a continuing dialogue with parliamentary, medical, professional and opinion-forming groups.

To get in touch with ISSUE, *see page 279.*

CHILD

CHILD and ISSUE are sister organisations working in very similar ways. Whilst they have been conducting exploratory talks about how they might work more closely together, a merger is not currently on the cards. They do of course collaborate on various campaigns to improve services for infertility nationwide through the NIAC (National Infertility Awareness Campaign). CHILD's main objective is to support infertile people through a combination of networking, information-giving and political campaigning. Its aims are:

- *To provide support,* counselling and information to those suffering the effects of infertility.
- *To encourage the exchange of information* and mutual support between couples themselves, for example by setting up local support groups.
- *To promote public awareness* as to the extent of infertility in the UK and the severe impact it can have on a couple's quality of life.

CHILD publish an excellent quarterly magazine with readers' stories, news and medical items, as well as a host of factsheets. They also run a 24-hour answering service called Linkline – for help, support, advice and a listening ear at any time and in strictest confidence.

Numerous UK clinics are affiliated to CHILD and members also have access to a broad selection of books which can be purchased via a discreet mail order. Their membership fee is £15 per annum (at time of writing).

To contact CHILD, *see page 279.*

Patient Support Groups

Most but not all clinics have Patient Support Groups. Some of these are run voluntarily and some have part- or full-time managers. Support groups are created by, for and with patients themselves and are therefore extremely varied. Some might concentrate on the social side, some on information-giving, others on campaigning. Prospect, which serves patients at the Hammersmith Hospital in London, actually succeeded in fundraising £18,000 in two years, a significant contribution to the costs of the new IVF Unit at Hammersmith Hospital. Tiffany Black, when with the ACU Patients Support Group at King's College Hospital in London, organised an Information Day in March 1996 attended by 400 people needing information about infertility. At the same time they also launched the National Egg Donation Campaign with hard-hitting posters, leaflets and advertising in the media. Some groups invite specialist speakers and have discussion evenings. All of them will have information, leaflets, addresses and books available to you. So there is a wide range of advantages to being part of a support group, and if you join one you can of course influence its activities. But many people find the idea of joining a group:

a) negative: 'If I join a group of infertiles I am confirming my infertility and what I really want to do is get pregnant/have a baby/think positive, not sit around moaning with fellow-sufferers.'

b) scary: 'what if I have to stand up and talk about myself in front of other people like they do in AA?'

Most people, if they do join a support group at all, will do so at the early stages of treatment as this can be a time of great stress and isolation. Once you are deeply involved in treatment cycles it is unlikely you will want to go to meetings. You might want to pledge your support instead by joining, paying the membership fee and staying in touch via their newsletter. Sometimes these newsletters publish writing by members – personal case stories, poems – and these can be both reassuring and touching to read. They also include news items, information about national campaigns, reviews of new books and the latest on current debates.

Contacts

If a group daunts you but you would like to keep in touch with people on an individual basis, you might seek informal contacts through CHILD and ISSUE or your Patient Support Group. You might be the sort of person who can easily connect with strangers and find the clinic waiting room an obvious place to make new friends. Don't be afraid of talking to people. You have a lot in common. They are also in pain. But don't be surprised if they aren't forthcoming. Some people really don't want to share what they are going through. If you do make new friendships through the clinic, bear in mind that the different outcome of your treatments can affect that relationship. It can be simply unbearable to know that your friend has succeeded where you have failed, or vice-versa. So keep an open mind and be honest with each other.

If a friend-of-a-friend has been through it all, don't be afraid of initiating contact. The worst response you can get is that they don't want to talk, but more often than not they will be happy to share their experiences. If you know of someone who has succeeded it can be encouraging, even inspiring, to see them whilst you are undergoing treatment. Fellow-infertiles often feel a real bond and understanding.

Like any minority, we have a very particular experience of life and exchanging stories can help make sense of the rollercoaster we've all been on.

(IV) Information Management: 'Coming Out' Infertile?

Every time we talk about infertility we make it easier for future couples to discuss.
CHRISSIE JONES, *THE EMOTIONAL SIDE OF INFERTILITY* (NEXT STEP PUBLISHING, 1995)

There are essentially two different ways to cope with your infertility crisis: to keep very quiet and private, only letting those really close to you know, or 'coming out' about what you are going through and converting your pain into a process of educating others and enlisting their support. Neither is right or wrong and you will choose which approach suits you best and helps you to remain in control. Let's briefly consider each option.

The 'Private' Way

You may have very good reasons for wishing or needing to keep quiet about what you are going through. You might know that

a) members of your family
b) colleagues
c) friends

won't

a) understand
b) support
c) accept

what you are going through. They may have strong ethical or religious objections, or they may have deep suspicions about the new technology. They might have a lot of anxiety. They may project this anxiety onto you. This is their problem, not yours. You might have the kind of relationship with these people which is strained or problematic in some way even without your infertility crisis. If that's the case, and you will know this better than anyone, then the choice not to tell them is very wise. If, however, you have really good relationships with these people, then your impulse not to tell might be to do with your own fear, guilt, shame or sense of failure. If that's so, think again. Confronting others with what you are going through might help to remove the stigma and anxiety. You can also train people to become your allies during this difficult phase of your life.

The important thing is to be very selfish and decide what really will work best for you in the long run. You might have to take some tough decisions, avoid people whom you love and who love you, even lie, but the main thing is that you take charge of your own support system and get all the help you need in the way that you want to receive it.

The 'Public' Way

Maria: *How can you say that?*

Yerma: *Because I'm sick and weary. Weary of being a woman not put to proper use. I'm hurt, hurt and humbled beyond endurance watching the crops springing up, the fountains flowing, the ewes bearing lambs and bitches their litter of pups, until it seems the whole countryside is teeming with mothers nursing their sleeping young. And here I am with two hammers beating at my breasts where my baby's mouth should be.*

Maria: *I hate to hear you talk like that.*

Yerma: *You mothers have no idea what it is like for us, any more than a swimmer in a mountain stream ever thinks of what it's like to be dying of thirst.*

FEDERICO GARCIA LORCA, *YERMA* (TRANS. PETER LUKE; METHUEN PLAYS, 1987)

The first step in going 'public' about your infertility is to find a way of talking about it. The second is choosing whom you tell and how. Only you will know how members of your family may react to the news that you or your partner are infertile and that you've chosen to undergo ART. When telling people, start by letting them know *what you are feeling.* This might pre-empt their feelings, which are not necessarily going to help you. Then explain how you've reached your decision and what the treatment process entails. Show them any literature you have on the subject. Draw diagrams. Let them know the timetable of your treatment cycle, the drugs and surgery, and be very clear as to how you would like them to show their support.

Telling colleagues may be hard but necessary. If you keep your treatment secret you may find yourself having to lie to get time off for medical appointments, and this duplicity can lead to feeling guilty or ashamed. On the other hand, you may not want everyone in your workplace to know what you're going through and you certainly don't want to encourage anybody's prejudice. One insensitive remark can make you feel lousy for a very long time after. You are in a hypersensitive state. On the surface you may be coping brilliantly and not letting anything slip or slide, but underneath you may be gripped by fear, misery and uncertainty.

I've always been very open about the fact that Sam was conceived through IVF. But it's easy to tell the whole world when you're safely pregnant or when you've given birth. When you're going through treatment you can actually feel very vulnerable, especially at work. When I was trying for a second baby, I confided in a handful of female colleagues with whom I worked closely rather than concoct elaborate stories to explain my absence from the office. I lived to regret it.

One day, when I was close to egg collection, I had to miss our weekly publishing meeting to go for a scan. I discovered that one of my trusted women colleagues, when asked where I was, had replied: 'Oh, she's off in hospital trying to get pregnant.' This in front of maybe 20 people, including male colleagues. People I liked, but with whom I would never have dreamed of discussing anything so intimate. My pain and humiliation were complete. The cycle was unsuccessful and I didn't have another try.
FREELANCE LITERARY EDITOR

So take a good look around you at work. Is there anyone you can trust to be understanding and discreet? Start with them. Explain what's happening and what you will need in the way of support. Gradually work your way round all those people you feel need to know so that you remain in control of the information. Why not write a schedule with the key days or times you need to take off work and give it to the relevant person or people? You could always ask your GP or your Consultant to supply you with a letter. This might help take the edge off the drama that can brew in other people's minds when they don't really understand something. It could help to make it all seem like an ordinary medical procedure. In short, don't internalise the stigma associated with infertility.

I always tell people that I have been infertile and that my son was conceived through IVF treatment. One of my friends said to me once: 'Why do you tell everyone, surely it is something to keep private?' I tell everyone though, because I'm so proud of it; of what I've been through and how I've come out the other end. I also think there might be someone listening who is going through the same thing and might need someone to talk to.
ROSEMARY HILL (TV PRODUCER)

If you do succeed in finding a way of managing information about your treatment which is clear, concise and gets people to understand your precise needs, you will not only have done yourself a huge service but will have helped educate the public in reaching a better understanding of Assisted Reproduction issues.

Whilst ART inhabits the public imagination only through sensationalist media stories and quotes from heavyweight medical experts, nothing will really change at a grass roots level. It is crucial that infertile people come forward and make known their situation, medically, socially and economically. A lot needs changing about ART in the UK. The first thing to change is people's minds. The rest, like all democratic social change, can only follow.

The magnitude of the issue of infertility does not present itself until each infertile individual declares the issue to themselves, and then others. We will never get society to accept infertility if we can't be honest about infertility to ourselves.
TIFFANY BLACK, ACU PATIENTS SUPPORT GROUP, KING'S COLLEGE HOSPITAL, LONDON, 1995

(v) Not Getting Pregnant/ Getting Pregnant

Not Getting Pregnant

You will probably have worked out before commencing any ART treatment how many attempts you will go for. Clinics differ in what they consider to be a healthy, wise and realistic number of treatment cycles. Some say that by the seventh IVF attempt a women usually conceives what has clumsily come to be known as a 'take-home baby', whilst others recommend sticking to around four attempts. Some people get addicted to trying and just can't stop. If you're an NHS patient the funding restrictions will of course determine your options. If you are paying privately and can see a way of funding your efforts *ad infinitum*, then you had probably best heed the advice of your doctors and tune in to your own body to pick up signals as to what it can endure.

Quitting

How do you come to terms with stopping, even when all your efforts haven't resulted in a baby? A friend of mine once said, after his partner miscarried at the age of 44: 'We've decided if we can't have a baby we'll have a BMW.' It was meant only half-ironically. Everybody will find their own substitutes for their dream child, and I don't feel it's my place to offer glib advice about how to come to terms with involuntary childlessness.

The important thing is to get rid of all notions of 'failure' in your mind. The word will probably have been bandied about a lot at the clinic. 'Failed cycle', 'failed fertilisation', 'failed attempt' are terms that get used all too frequently and can penetrate deep in the psyche.

When you've undergone infertility treatment which hasn't proved successful, you have at least taken an active role in reaching the conclusion that a child (or another child) won't happen 'naturally' for you. For many people this is a preferred option than never having ventured along the ART path. You will have gone on a steep learning curve medically, emotionally, ethically and psychologically. Your relationship will have been buffeted from all sides. Some couples never fully recover from the blows. If your relationship has weathered the storms it may be stronger than ever. You will now have the rest of your life and your options to consider. Perhaps you will research adoption – from the UK, or maybe from abroad (*see Chapter 6*). Whatever you decide, it will doubtlessly be easier than the endless cliffhanging during your infertility treatment.

There are compensations for childlessness, of course there are, even though it is so impossible to see them when you are consumed with trying to make a baby. Now is the time to concentrate on those advantages, the most significant being your freedom.

Getting Pregnant

When they had finished their simple meal of rice and dried fish, Grandmama cleaned the big kitchen knife. Together they put their hands on the haft and gently sliced down the golden cleft of the peach. As it fell apart, there was a stirring in the heart of the fruit. They fell back in fear as a boy, gay as the first green of spring, stepped out before their astounded eyes.
THE PEACH BOY, JAPANESE TALES AND LEGENDS (EDS HELEN AND WILLIAM MCALPINE; OXFORD UNIVERSITY PRESS, 1958)

If you've achieved a pregnancy through ART you will be feeling over the moon and probably incredulous that after everything you've gone through there actually is a baby (or babies) growing inside. You now have to make the transition from being an infertility patient to being a pregnant woman, and that isn't as easy as it may sound. For one thing, the clinic will encourage caution in the first few weeks to make absolutely sure that the pregnancy isn't ectopic and that you don't miscarry (around 14.6 per cent of clinical pregnancies after IVF miscarry). You may also find that your whole psyche continues to be so full of the ART experience it's really hard to let go and confidently join the ranks of the antenatal mums.

The hospital environment itself might contribute to your alienation. Antenatal classes can be cosy affairs, full of either very young women or older women with a brood already in tow. If you are older and this pregnancy is your first, you may feel a bit of a prune. If you opt for extra-mural preparation you may find your Active Birth teacher crowing about the lovely natural things you can do with your body in preparation for a dreamy, aromatherapy-drenched birth-pool delivery, when you suspect or know you will be having a Caesarean. Other women might make all kinds of assumptions and be quite oblivious to what you've gone through. You may dread the moment when you are asked to talk about your pregnancy to the group when everyone else seems to have got a bun in the oven from merely sitting on the loo after their partner. You may be acutely reminded of the 'unnatural' process by which you got your own 'bump'.

The point is, you are in a minority and have to live with that. You might decide to keep quiet about how you became pregnant, or you may want to gently use the situation of antenatal culture to consciousness-raise amongst the fertile. Whatever you do, don't feel bad or let any of the fertile world's ignorance blemish the joy of your own hard-won pregnancy.

There may be a lot of pressure on you to be in a constant state of ecstasy. Your friends, family and loved ones will be 'so happy for you' and won't necessarily understand that during your pregnancy you may, just like any other woman, feel ill, daunted, tired, depressed, deflated and confused. You may feel churlish not going round with a permanent grin plastered across your face, and may find it really hard just to BE PREGNANT rather than BE HAVING A MIRACLE PREGNANCY.

Then you will have the worry of tests to undergo, and the added fear that 'something may be wrong' with your precious cargo. You wouldn't be the first person to encounter medical staff during your antenatal care who continue to refer to your fertility treatment and how 'precious' your 'IVF baby' or babies are. The point is, nobody means harm and of course your pregnancy is miraculous and special – but then every baby is a miracle. Don't forget, science and technology only created the conditions. It was you and Nature who made it all happen.

Come the birth there may be reasons why a Caesarean section is recommended. It could be a factor of age, or that the baby (or babies) are in a breech position, or the fact you are expecting twins or triplets (in which case you will have been admitted to hospital earlier on in your pregnancy). A C-section might be advised when there is any real risk to you and the baby, and you may well hear medics saying 'after all, this is an IVF pregnancy.' So what do you do? It is 'an IVF pregnancy' (or DI or ICSI or whatever). It is also YOUR PREGNANCY and nobody else's. You need to try and refocus. You have spent months, perhaps years, in a highly clinical setting undergoing very invasive medical treatment. You are now a prospective mother (and father). You need to try and tune in to what's going on inside and get on with preparing to have your baby in the best possible way.

Your baby (babies) are born. This might have been under water, on a bed, squatting on the floor or lying on your back full of drugs whilst the doctors removed it from you surgically. However it happens, a little tiny dependent creature(s) is now yours. Everyone around you will probably continue to expect you to float on Cloud 9, as well you might. The reality is, you are now just an ordinary mum of a newborn infant. You will be exhausted from lack of sleep, your relationship will undergo a momentous transformation and be tested to the limit, you will be coping with dirty nappies, feeding rituals and adjustment to the enormity of the birth event. Somewhere in all of this cluttering and clamouring you may well just want to cry, be depressed, be 'copeless' (just like any other new mum) and may find it impossible to let anyone know how you are feeling in case you appear ungrateful. My own partner wrote at the time:

July 21: The baby is more than a month old now. Anna has been going round with a permanent smile on her face. I gave her a real talking to about that today. 'Complain,' I begged. She clearly feels that there was so much pressure on me to have this baby that she's not allowed ever to say anything negative whatsoever. It's a touching thought, but she's about to blow up, taking the street with her.

'JACK KLAFF'S IVF DIARY'. THE *GUARDIAN*, 3RD APRIL 1996

Well, a little bit of postnatal depression might well be hormonal. It doesn't mean you are the inconsolable Tsarina to whom no amount of Fabergé eggs can bring joy. The point is you have become 'normal' after so long a period of feeling deviant and alienated. A pregnancy rushes by. You may not have had time to adjust. You need time, you need space and you need to communicate how you are feeling without guilt or shame. Above all, you need to concentrate on your child(ren) and how fantastic they are and what a brilliant thing you all did in getting this far.

CHAPTER (4)

Access

i. Funding Your Treatment

① Funding Your Treatment

A mother who stole £20,000 from her employers to pay for IVF treatment escaped jail after a judge took mercy on her. The case of Michelle Darby (27) who received a 12-month sentence suspended for two years, must have struck a chord with many women who are desperate for children.
OLDHAM EVENING CHRONICLE, 17TH APRIL 1996

Is an end to the postcode lottery in sight?
At the time of writing there is positive news to report. Years of campaigning to achieve better funding appears, at last, to be having some effect in government thinking. On 30th November 2000, the Secretary for State for Health in England, Alan Milburn, issued a press release entitled 'Working Towards Ending the Postcode Lottery of Infertility Treatment'. In it he announced that he would be asking the National Institute of Clinical Excellence (NICE) to consider and update existing clinical guidelines issued by the Royal College of Obstetricians and Gynaecologists (RCOG). This endorsement of national guidelines is a significant first for the NHS. The statement goes on to mention the survey published that day showing unequivocally the 'postcode lottery' system at work given that some health authorities are currently spending £500,000 a year on treatments whilst others are spending none.

Milburn stated:

That postcode lottery has to end now, given the scale of extra resources we are putting into the NHS ... In the future I see no reason why new drug treatments should not comprise a much higher share of the rising NHS budget ... NICE epitomises the philosophy which lies at the heart of the NHS; care based on patients' clinical need, not on their ability to pay or where they happen to live.

CHILD and NIAC welcomed the news with cautious optimism. Clare Brown of CHILD issued the following statement in a press release 30th November 2000:

I hope that Health Authorities in England, Wales and Northern Ireland will not waste time waiting for the NICE guidance, start reviewing what they currently provide and begin to address local provision as soon as possible before too much more valuable fertile time is wasted.

whilst Berkeley Greenwood, political advisor to NIAC wrote in a response for *CHILDchat*:

NICE will need to decide under what circumstances particular treatments such as IVF and ICSI should be provided and when it would not be appropriate to use them. This process could take as long as a year. It may be decided that IVF and ICSI should be used only restrictively and the challenge for all those campaigning for infertility is to collect and submit the strongest possible arguments to support the use of these modern treatments ... We also need to bear two facts in mind. Both Ministers and priorities do change and, furthermore, whilst the idea of making funding available for infertility has been hinted at, it has not yet been promised and nor is it clear where it will come from.

Against the indication that funding for fertility treatment might undergo a shake-up in the foreseeable future, and assuming that restrictions and conditions for access to treatment will still prevail, it is worth considering the funding situation currently in force, how it functions within the re-structuring of the NHS undertaken by the Tories, and how this reflects attitudes to infertility in general:

The current picture

Nowhere has the stigma of infertility been more keenly felt than in the UK's totally inequitable NHS funding schemes. There is currently no national policy for NHS provision. Instead, each Health Authority decides its own policy and the criteria within it. Virginia Bottomley's Patient's Charter clearly states:

*You have the **right** to:*
Receive health care on the basis of your clinical need, not on your ability to pay, your lifestyle or any other factor;
NHS PATIENT'S CHARTER, DEPT OF HEALTH, JANUARY 1995

but because infertility is not seen as a 'clinical need' (illness) it doesn't apply. The low status infertility treatment is given throughout the NHS is borne out by the Charter going on to state:

In March 1991 over 50,000 patients were waiting 2 years or more to go in to hospital. Now nobody waits this long (except for a handful of patients waiting for specialist fertility treatment).

Those in charge of the NHS are operating a rationing scheme, euphemistically disguised by the term 'priority setting'. Across the board, these 'priorities', say the Government, should be determined by doctors, and whilst the Government may issue guidelines, these are not, say the Ministers, 'instructions'. To use the analogy of a menu, the Government neither decides what is on the menu, nor what doctors should choose from it. But the Government is inconsistent in this, and the national mess of funding infertility treatment is a case in point. With IVF, the decision of what might be 'on the menu' (if indeed anything should be on it at all) is left to the Health Authorities; clinicians select from this. Thus menus are being devised at a local rather than a national level, with ludicrously complicated knock-on effects for patients. Put quite simply, your access to treatment on the NHS will depend on where you live combined with your personal circumstances, assessed both by doctors and bureaucrats in local government. Is this lottery really a '*National* Health Service'? Wasn't the post-war commitment to the NHS precisely a pledge to eliminate all discussions thenceforth about whom should get treatment and by what criteria?

Politicians cannot assess who should receive treatment and how much they should get. Pragmatism dictates that this must be left to clinicians. But only politicians can decide what has to be paid for and what not.
BILL NEW AND JULIAN LE GRAND, *RATIONING AND THE NHS: PRINCIPLES AND PRAGMATISM* (FROM THE KING'S FUND, AS QUOTED IN THE *GUARDIAN*, 24TH JULY 1996)

People in (local) authority are making judgements about infertility in order to make judgements about provision, and refusal for treatment is mainly done on social rather than medical grounds. G. B. Shaw may well have said:

Parentage is a very important profession, but no test of fitness for it is ever imposed in the interest of the children.
EVERYBODY'S POLITICAL WHAT'S WHAT (1944)

but he never lived long enough to witness the Local Health Authorities (LHAs), guided by legislation and/or ignorance, use this idea for outright discrimination against thousands of citizens who simply can't reproduce without medical help. Where the fertile population have access to abortion and sterilisation (costing much the same as an IVF cycle), the infertile have to jump through hoops to justify their very ordinary quest for a child of their own.

Currently 90 per cent of IVF treatment is in the private sector in the UK. Compare this figure with provision in other countries: France, where up to four cycles of IVF are provided free, Germany up to four, Belgium up to three and Australia up to six.

The dire picture of NHS funding for infertility treatment led Jenny Murray to the apt question on BBC's Women's Hour (17th July 1996),

Can only 'nice' people have babies?

Infertility treatment is a gamble and the stakes are high. You are investing your hopes, your body and very often your own money into what may be a less than one in four chance of success. I have heard of people mortgaging their homes, moving house to live in a providing Authority, passing the hat round at work, and of course praying for a Lottery win to pay for the chance of making a baby. There is something deeply unpleasant – even offensive – about having to think about money in connection with the creation of a new life. But in our cash-card society even matters of life and death themselves have become subject to price tags and economy drives.

The ease with which the message spoken by involuntary childlessness has been translated into the language of consumerism is in keeping with the politically driven tendency that emerged in the late 1980s, through which all medical encounters are being converted into market transactions: patients are customers now.

NAOMI PFEFFER, *THE STORK AND THE SYRINGE* (POLITY PRESS, 1993)

For some of you reading this book, funding treatment yourself is out of the question. What can you do? You must try every avenue of obtaining NHS funding, and if that fails you have the option to campaign and appeal. More of that later. Before discussing how to find your way round the complexity of funding, let's put the current situation into context:

The Effect on Your Chances of Treatment

The problems of waiting, not for treatment, but for funding for treatment. What does one do after that one cycle? Self fund? that option is not open to all. Wait for a change in funding policy? That change might not come soon enough.

JACQUELINE PASCHOUD (CHAIR, ACU PATIENT SUPPORT GROUP, KING'S COLLEGE HOSPITAL, LONDON), *KING'S UPDATE: THE NEWSLETTER OF THE KING'S ACU SUPPORT GROUP*, SPRING 1996

In major health reforms introduced in 1989 and management restructuring, the Conservative government concentrated on turning hospitals into Trusts (providers) and Health Authorities into purchasers with a responsibility towards their patient population (consumers) who, apparently, have 'choice'. Since its 'corporitisation' our Health Service is described in the language of business, and competitiveness is actively encouraged. The annual NHS Comparative Performance ('League') Tables were published for the first time in June 1994, showing how local hospitals and emergency services are doing against some national standards. This whole shake-up deliberately created an internal market, with hospitals competing with each other to provide services, each bidding to their Local Health Authority for funds within an overall climate of reduced funding. This in turn has put an emphasis on a 'value for money' ethos on the part of Health Authorities and a pressure on hospitals to produce 'results'. In such a climate certain services have been reduced, particularly those, such as plastic surgery and fertility treatment, which are considered a luxury, not a necessity.

Biological dysfunctions which are socially debilitating, such as deafness,
are certainly regarded as the proper business of medicine to cure or alleviate.
It is indeed ironic that health planning policies will make resources available
to reduce the biological dysfunction of sterility in men and women for clinical
and social reasons when they will not invest in services to resolve such
dysfunctions.

DONALD EVANS, *INTRODUCTION TO CREATING THE CHILD – THE ETHICS, LAW AND*
PRACTICE OF ASSISTED CONCEPTION (MARTINUS NIJHOFF PUBLISHERS, 1996)

It might not surprise you to know that infertility is not considered an
illness. It may anger you that factors such as your statistical chances of
success based on, for example, your age, will play their part in Health
Authorities' decisions. It may appal you to know that Health Authorities
are far from uniform in their funding policies regarding what treatments
they will fund, if any. For instance, whilst 52 per cent of District Health
Authorities currently provide some IVF on the NHS, 48 per cent do not.[1]

If you are 'lucky' enough to live within a Health Authority that does fund
treatment, you may find all manner of potential obstacles to your goals.
Some Authorities may fund drug treatment but not IVF and its variants.
Some may fund tubal surgery but not IVF. Some may only offer IVF provided
you are married and childless (even if any child you have was from a former
relationship). Most have an upper age limit of anything between 30 and 35
years. These age limits are based on statistics and driven by the 'League
Table' ethos. It is a statistical fact that the success rate for IVF drops by a few
percent after the age of 35, and that by 40+ a woman's chances of achieving
a pregnancy may be as little as 5–9 per cent. The older woman is therefore
seen by NHS funders as a waste of money. The fact remains that a working
woman of 40 has paid 10 more years' taxes and by any other criteria such
as financial and emotional stability might prove herself entirely suitable
for treatment.

[Older] women have delayed childbearing until they've developed their skills.
They're likely to be more mature, maybe better parents. By their contribution
to society they've more than paid their NHS treatment.

PROFESSOR ROBERT WINSTON, *EVENING STANDARD*, 2ND APRIL 1996

Hospitals and District Health Authorities/Providers and Purchasers

The Health Service has a 'vertical' structure. Money is provided by the Government to the Department of Health which is then passed down to the Health Authorities. These were previously divided into District Health Authorities and Family Health Service Authorities, but since 1st April 1996 have merged to become Local Health Authorities (LHAs).

> Figures for NHS spending on IVF are not held centrally but estimated at approximately £25 million annually.

One of the unfortunate side-effects of health reforms is an over-bureaucratisation of the system. You may well be affected by this in your quest for NHS-funded treatment.

How LHAs May Fund a Licensed NHS or Private Clinic: Block Contracts and Extra-contractual Referrals (ECRs)

Block Contracts

A block contract is an agreement to treat a set number of patients per year within an agreed set of criteria. If patients fit these criteria, they go on a waiting list. On the whole it is a much faster process than ECRs and gives the clinic more power in assessing the patients' criteria.

Extra-contractual Referrals

Here the clinic or GP applies to the LHA for each patient per treatment cycle. Application forms present no diagnostic information nor case history, so in effect the LHA has only the most rudimentary information on which to base its decision.

Most Authorities operate on an ECR basis because it offers much tighter control over spending and the procedure gives the LHA more power to assess the criteria. This also means that the funding is dependent on whether or not the LHA has already spent its allocation for individual treatments for the year in which you are applying.

In cases where the patient seeks treatment from a hospital outside his or her own LHA, an ECR would automatically be applied for from a budget the LHA has set aside for any treatments (not only infertility) that it can't provide locally.

The time scale between applying for an ECR and response from the LHA is generally up to three months.

The Role of Your GP

The funding situation on the NHS is further complicated by the role of your GP. LHAs won't always automatically include the cost of drugs in your treatment, and hospitals would prefer you to get these through your GP rather than to be eating into their own stressed drug budget. A GP's decision on whether or not to supply you with a prescription may in turn be more to do with the practice's own financial considerations than any ethical ones. Drugs can be extremely costly. Ampoules of ovary-stimulating drugs cost about £10 each, and patients may need anything between 30 to 100 or more per treatment cycle.

If you are going through NHS-funded treatment and your GP refuses to supply you with drugs, you can either change GPs or contact your IVF Unit and tell them of your situation. The Hospital Business Manager (or equivalent) may be able to arrange for the LHA to cover the costs separately.

It can help your GP to decide on whether to give you the drugs on prescription if you can support your request with a letter from your Consultant explaining your diagnosis, proposed treatment and information about the drugs you are to be prescribed. Your GP may, however, be prevented from prescribing the drugs because his or her LHA has a policy against it. It is worth contacting your LHA to find out. You are entitled to argue that this policy limits your access to treatment.

Ares-Serono, the Swiss pharmaceuticals group that specialise in human fertility drugs yesterday reported a 4.1 per cent increase in net profit last year to $29.4 million from $28.2 million in 1994 ... group sales of infertility products which rose 10 per cent in 1995 were expected to show double-digit growth annually for the next 5 years.
FINANCIAL TIMES, 22ND MARCH 1996

Drugs purchased via the GP/local pharmacy route may cost the taxpayer more than twice what they would cost via the hospital pharmacy. So the fall-out of efficiency drives and book-balancing within an underfunded system is actually an increase in costs to the taxpayer. Professor Winston of the Hammersmith Hospital estimates that such mismanagement of resources actually costs the NHS an extra £5 million a year, or 'enough to give another 5,000 patients one chance at IVF on an NHS basis in NHS Hospitals'.[11]

The Hidden Costs of Infertility Treatment

A shopworker who was sacked after taking time off for fertility treatment lost her case for sexual discrimination yesterday.
DARLINGTON NORTHERN ECHO, 19TH MARCH 1996

It is worth considering some of the hidden costs you will meet. This will definitely include *time*, *travel* and, if you work, certainly *time off work*. You will also have to face some *emotional cost* and a great deal of *stress* which might lead to *exhaustion*, *depression* and *anxiety*. If you are put on an NHS waiting list you might have to wait a long time for treatment, and this could put an immense *strain* on you and your relationship. It is easier to calculate the practical costs than the emotional ones, but it is worth sitting down with your partner and making a realistic list of these and other 'hidden' costs when weighing up your options.

We as counsellors must be alert to people who are putting themselves beyond their resources, and I don't just mean financial. I'm talking in terms of energy, emotions and time.
REVEREND TIM APPLETON, INFERTILITY COUNSELLOR, *OLDHAM EVENING CHRONICLE*,
17TH APRIL 1996

If You Are Refused NHS Funding

Some NHS clinics will treat you at the cost-price to a Health Authority (such as approximately £800 for an IVF cycle, as compared to the normal £1,000 – £2,000). Basically hospitals which do this aren't making a profit from patients but helping the more needy have access to treatment. Hospitals get drugs more cheaply than community pharmacies, so if your LHA and GP both refuse to pay for your drugs, it is advisable to purchase them at the clinic.

You may wish to appeal against the decision by writing a personal letter to The Chief Executive of your LHA (her/his name will be available from your GP or NHS Hospital), outlining your case history in detail. Often LHAs refuse treatment more through ignorance than wilful obstruction, and may in certain cases revoke their decision when they have a more complete picture. This may be particularly so in cases, for instance, where a woman's age falls just outside their stated age limit. If you have the energy it is well worth trying. Let your Hospital's Business Manager know you want to do this, and get his or her support as well as that of your Patient Support Group if there is one. The National Infertility Awareness Campaign (NIAC), ISSUE and CHILD will also help and will be interested in receiving copies of any replies you receive.

Some questions to ask your Local Health Authority about their current and strategic plans for infertility investigation and treatment:

- What investigations do you provide for people with an infertility problem? for example:
  - laparoscopy?
  - ultrasound scans?
  - blood tests?
  - full semen analysis?
- Will drugs such as gonadotrophins be available?
- Do you provide treatments such as IVF and GIFT? (If not, do you intend to contract with another Health Authority or private clinic to provide these treatments – and if so, which?)
- Do you intend to ration these treatments – and if so, how?
- Do you provide (or contract with another Health Authority or private clinic to provide) tubal surgery?

NIAC recommends that when writing to the Authorities you stress that, although fertility treatment is perceived as having a relatively low success rate, in fact the 'normal' conception rate is only 20–25 per cent a month. So an IVF treatment with a pregnancy success rate of 25 per cent should be compared to this figure. Also, tell them that investing in infertility treatment is investing in the future of our society. You might also alert them to the hidden costs of infertility to the NHS in terms of, for example, GPs' time, counselling, and the social cost.

Health Authorities are public bodies and are required to be responsive to public pressure. It is your right to appeal against a decision they have made on your behalf. If this still fails, and you still have the fighting spirit, write to your local MP (you can get her or his name from your local library). MPs tend to have close dealings with Health Authorities as well as being in a position to talk to Ministers.

Remember, you are not alone! Get the support you need. The National Infertility Awareness Campaign (*see below*) is involved in trying to improve people's right for a family of their own, as are organisations such as ISSUE and CHILD (*see page 279*). One of the painful ironies of infertility is that at the very moment when you might be best poised to turn your private experience into a campaign for your rights as a citizen, you are probably going to be feeling depressed, isolated and powerless. You may be going through real despair at having funding refused, and grief at your childlessness in a very private way, and consequently find it very hard to summon the energy and motivation to fight for your own, let alone other people's, rights. This is perfectly understandable, but you do need to know your options, where to get the help you need and what kind of work is going on to help people in your predicament. After all, by 'coming out' of our shame and our pain, by standing up and being counted, by working together and forcing the issues out into the open, we can hope to achieve a fairer system for all.

The National Infertility Awareness Campaign (NIAC)

This is an umbrella organisation for its supporters, who include organisations, clinics and colleges, Patient Support Groups and international organisations. They have all pledged their support for NIAC's objectives, which are:

- to convince Health Ministers and Officials that more modern and cost-effective investigation and treatment should be routinely offered by Health Authorities in preference to older treatments which have lower success rates
- to achieve a full range of infertility investigations and treatments throughout the country, together with a uniform provision, given that fertile couples have access in each LHA to most types of treatment from contraception to birth and beyond
- to communicate their five key messages to the public, LHAs, MPs and the Department of Health through patients and professionals involved in infertility.

NIAC's five key messages are:

1. One in six couples seek medical help in order to achieve pregnancy.
2. Couples who are denied access to appropriate treatment face profound psychological and emotional strain.
3. Excellent results can be achieved in treating infertility if the patient is rapidly investigated and referred for appropriate treatment.
4. To delay referral or progression of patients to the appropriate treatment reduces the likelihood of success.
5. The chance of conception in any one month for an average fertile couple is 20–25 per cent. The success rate for infertility treatment should be set against this base line.

To contact NIAC, *see Useful Addresses.*

If you are paying for your treatment yourself, always be sure to find out what the price being quoted to you covers. For example, does it include drugs? counselling? blood tests? anaesthetic? etc. If not, write a list, with the clinic, of every single thing your treatment will involve and the itemised cost of each.

Criteria for Funding and Treatment: Being Assessed

A heartbroken woman claims she was taken off a fertilisation course after experts found her husband had been in prison.
GLASGOW HERALD, 19TH MARCH 1996

Current legislation in the UK means that in seeking Assisted Conception you have to make public a very intimate and natural desire. This desire for a child will not be taken for granted by either funders nor many doctors, and your access to treatment will depend on both medical and social factors. Whilst 'fertiles' can choose to breed in privacy, infertiles have to justify why they want a child and what their personal circumstances might be. This process might not be obvious to you, particularly if your social circumstances conform more to the traditional norm. But whether or not you 'pass' will affect your chances of both treatment and funding. You might be forgiven for assuming that if you go private you will have instant purchasing power, but even this isn't necessarily so. Doctors make their own judgements as to whether or not they want to treat certain patients based on the medical picture before them and their obligation by law to consider the welfare of any child born by their medical intervention. But how can a doctor predict and judge the future in this way? And how can capricious or prejudiced decisions by doctors be prevented? Some have been known to have their own hidden agendas for refusing to treat a patient. These are hard to prove (for example if a patient is considered 'difficult') whilst the majority have an open policy to refuse treatment to single women or lesbian couples. Should the ultimate power of infertility consultants be reined in by forcing their hospital's ethics committee to be consulted? Ethics committees include laypeople, and exist precisely to help doctors with some of the knottier decisions regarding treatment, but many hospitals don't have these committees and there is no uniform policy on how to use them. In reality, therefore, individual consultants wield enormous power over infertile people's lives.

An artificial, intense relationship is created between a woman (almost always) and a doctor (usually male) which frequently makes major demands on finance, and puts great stress on family and couple relationships. This relationship is also highly dependent, with the 'patient' often regressing into

being 'the good child' in order for the omnipotent doctor/father or clinical
spouse to overcome the lack of fertility or potential for impregnation ... people
have to pay for something which other people in society have gratis. Each
setting sets up a kind of blueprint ... of the ideal type of person who should be
allowed for treatment.

SUE EMMY JENNINGS, 'THE HEALING POWER OF THE DRAMATIZED HERE AND NOW',
IN *DRAMATIC APPROACHES TO BRIEF DRAMATHERAPY* (ED. ALIDA GERSIE;
JESSICA KINGSLEY, 1995)

Two major factors can affect a doctor's decision to treat you: First, League
Tables. These mean that clinics might reject a 'risky' patient so that their
success rates look good, thus discriminating against patients with a more
complicated prognosis. League tables are commercially motivated and, in
Professor Winston's view, lead to unscrupulousness '... people will lie about
the results. Standards will go down, not up, and it will be the infertile
couple that suffers.'[III] Secondly: legislation as set out in the HFEA guidelines.
One of the stated conditions of a treatment licence is that:

A woman shall not be provided with treatment services unless account has
been taken of the welfare of any child who may be born as a result of the
treatment (including the need of that child for a father) and of any other child
who may be affected by the birth.

THE HUMAN FERTILISATION AND EMBRYOLOGY ACT 1990 S 13(5)

The HFEA Code of Practice goes on to list the following factors which licensed
clinics should bear in mind when assessing patients' suitability for treatment:

a) their commitment to having and bringing up a child or children
b) their ability to provide a stable and supportive environment for any child
   produced as a result of treatment
c) their medical histories and the medical histories of their families
d) their ages and likely future ability to look after or provide for a child's needs
e) their ability to meet the needs of any child or children who may be born
   as a result of treatment, including the implications of any possible
   multiple births
f) any risk of harm to the child or children who may be born, including the
   risk of inherited disorders, problems during pregnancy and of neglect or
   abuse
g) the effect of a new baby or babies upon any existing child of the family.[IV]

Now, the above qualifications for parenting, if applied throughout society, might be an excellent way of improving the welfare of all children born and preventing the plight of unwanted, neglected and abused children. As it is, applying these screening processes only to infertile adults is unjust. In a recent book about infertility, the authors lump together various 'marginals' – alcoholics, drug-users, child abusers, the mentally ill, prostitutes and those who are HIV positive – as undesirable for treatment. This list reveals an overt link between assessment and bias. Whilst anyone with a record of committing child abuse clearly has a disturbed and potentially dangerous attitude towards children, which would almost certainly disqualify them for Assisted Conception, why should women who work as prostitutes not have children of their own? Prostitution is a job, not a personality disorder. As for lesbian couples, there is no evidence to suggest that children brought up in loving, stable, single-sex relationships are disadvantaged. Yet the fact that the HFEA doesn't favour lesbians as potential mothers is implied in the statement 'including the need of that child for a father'.[v] The recent case of a patient with HIV treated by Professor Winston at the Hammersmith Hospital hit the headlines after an episode of the BBC's *Making Babies*, in which Professor Winston was arguing his case with his team. The subject is clearly emotive, and the 'welfare of the child' was foremost in the minds of some of his team members, who had concerns about treating this patient. Professor Winston's argument was essentially ethical: If he were to discriminate against a patient who might contract AIDS in the near future, how come there is no moral objection to the treatment of patients with terminal cancer or those who know they carry the gene for a fatal disease, meaning their baby has a 50/50 chance of inheriting it?

I have no idea whether Sheila with her HIV infection, or indeed any of my patients, will make good parents. In fact, I am not sure whether I would qualify for that accolade myself. What troubles me most about this arbitrary process, whereby we impose our values on other people – often perhaps those who are less articulate, knowledgeable, or well provided than ourselves – is that we are in a position to do so simply because they are suffering from a disease process. No other free member of society is vetted before he or she decides that they want to have a baby.

PROFESSOR ROBERT WINSTON, *MAKING BABIES* (BBC BOOKS, 1993)

Finally, one of the most worrying things about the combination of the HFEA's Code of Practice concerning the patient and the haphazard and fragmented way in which funding decisions are made nationally is that it effectively privileges the rich and victimises the poor and the marginalised. And that, quite simply, is why it is important for patients to demand their rights, to question authority and to work towards a fairer deal for all. You may not have the stamina to do so whilst you are in the midst of treatment. You may be focusing all your energies on your own baby-making goals. But don't forget that whatever you might go through in funding your treatment, YOU ARE NOT ALONE.

NHS Organisations: Who Controls Whom?

How money for your treatment comes into the control of the Health Authorities:

Secretary of State for Health
Department of Health
NHS Policy Board
NHS Executive
Regional Offices

Health Authorities*   NHS Trusts Hospitals
Community Health Councils/GPs
Dentists/Opticians/Retail Pharmacists

* Before April 1996, Health Authorities were divided into District Health Authorities and Family Health Service Authorities.

How to Go About Getting NHS Funding

Your GP

refers you to

A LOCAL HOSPITAL

refers you to

A SPECIALIST FERTILITY CLINIC

confirms your subfertility and accepts you for specific treatment

NB: YOU TAKE ACTION NOW *by calling*

YOUR LOCAL HEALTH AUTHORITY
to find out their criteria and whether you and your required treatment fit them

if 'yes'	*if 'no'*
The HOSPITAL *and* HEALTH AUTHORITY	*if a) you are not eligible*
will make an application on your behalf.	*b) your required treatment*
	isn't funded you can
You will go on a	
WAITING LIST	
NB: APPLY NOW TO YOUR GP for drugs,	APPEAL TO THE LHA
supported by a letter from the	*a) with support from the clinic*
Fertility Clinic.	*b) without support*
	writing an outline of your
	case history
	if still 'no':
	WRITE TO YOUR MP
	Remember:
	GET SUPPORT *from doctors,*
	support groups and campaign
	organisations.

CHAPTER (5)

Alternatives to High-tech Reproduction

i. Complementary Medicine and Self-help

After a time of decay comes the turning point. The powerful light that has been banished returns. There is movement, but it is not brought about by force ... The movement is natural, arising spontaneously. For this reason the transformation of the old becomes easy. The old is discarded and the new is introduced. Both measures accord with the time; therefore no harm results.
FROM THE *I-CHING*

① Complementary Medicine and Self-help

The word 'patient' is revealing. It stems from the Latin word *patientia*, meaning 'suffering' or 'endurance'. To 'be patient' is to remain passive-in-waiting. To be 'a patient' is to be 'long-suffering' or 'one who endures'. Waiting passively for a long time may well be exactly what you find yourself expected to do when undergoing infertility treatment. This chapter hopes to show you how to become more pro-active in your treatment process, how to help yourself and how to find ways to balance the rigours of drugs, surgery and other highly invasive forms of medical treatment with other, more ancient methods.

During the past 400 years, Western science has become obsessed with measurement and quantification. Before 1500, people lived in a world in which the universe was perceived as organic and spiritual. God, Nature and Humanity's quest for knowledge were seen as harmonious, and the goal of science was to interpret rather than to control things. The 17th century saw a revolution in the history of Western civilisation. In his work *Discourse on the Method of Rightly Conducting One's Reason and Searching the Truth in the Sciences*, the French philosopher René Descartes declared his famous theory: *Cogito, ergo sum* ('I think, therefore I am'), introducing the idea that 'Man' could reason deductively and analytically, and, crucially, that Mind was separate from Matter: 'there is nothing included in the concept of body that belongs to the mind; and nothing in that mind that belongs to the body.' This mind-body split has continued to dominate our whole culture.[1] Descartes used the metaphor of a clock to describe the human body:

'I consider the human body as a machine ... my thought ... compares a sick man and an ill-made clock with my idea of a healthy man and a well-made clock.' It is not hard to see how his views have continued to influence Western medicine. In Western medicine the human body is broken down into its component parts, and the sick 'bits' are treated, usually in isolation. Disease is 'attacked' with drugs or 'cut out' with surgery, and the doctor remains the active, expert and powerful God in whom we invest our ignorant faith.

Nowhere is this more true than in the field of infertility. The Specialist Consultant decides our fate from the start by accepting to treat us or not; we then invest this person with almost magical power to fulfil our dreams. Drugs like suppressing or superovulation hormones are used to shut down or accelerate the body's natural tempos, other hormones to 'kickstart' the system, whilst the use of microsurgery has introduced the idea of breaking problems down into smaller and smaller units to the point where, assisted by technology, we are able to 'see' images of our own reproductive cells which in reality are so small the mind can barely imagine them. It is easy to collaborate in this process of fragmentation, to stop experiencing your body as a whole and visualise it instead as 'bits' which don't 'work' or are 'a problem'.

The whole field of ART depends on isolating such 'problems' and examining them in vastly magnified detail. It is certainly a boon to infertile people everywhere that Western, deductive scientific research has led to the technique of isolating the minute single sperm and egg and introducing them to each other. But where does that leave the 'patient' and what can we do to remain integrated and connected meanwhile?

Complementary medicine might not necessarily 'cure' you. It can't, for instance, repair a damaged tube or replace an absent uterus. It can, however, work alongside your mainstream treatment to help balance out your system, to strengthen you, to relax you and to make you feel more healthy, positive and in control of your own body. In recent years there has been a proliferation of alternative medical practices now generally called 'complementary' because they can be used to complement, or support, mainstream treatment. There isn't room in this book to cover them all, but the following represent some of the most common and respected.

Chinese Medicine

In Western medicine the doctor with the highest reputation is a specialist who has detailed knowledge about a specific part of the body. In Chinese medicine, the ideal doctor is a sage who knows how all the patterns of the universe work together; who treats each patient on an individual basis; whose diagnosis does not categorise the patient as having a specific disease but records as fully as possible the individual's total state of mind and body and its relation to the natural and social environment.

FRITJOF CAPRA, *THE TURNING POINT* (FLAMINGO, 1983)

The Chinese idea of the body is concerned with the interrelationship of its parts rather than anatomical accuracy. Thus, in both male and female infertility, the organ associated with any dysfunction would be the kidneys (which are believed to store all inherited functions) and treatment would involve strengthening the 'kidney function' – that is, the function the kidney performs in the body's entire system. This system of interrelating parts is kept harmonious by a system of dynamic balance between what is known as *yin* (the 'feminine') and *yang* (the 'masculine') qualities. Whilst going in and out of balance is seen as a natural process and part of the life-cycle, illness or dysfunction is seen as an imbalance of yin or yang in any part or parts of the body as a whole which can, through treatment, be rebalanced. Central to this process of balance is the concept of energy flowing through the body – or *'chi. 'Chi* is not a substance but a flow of energy. This flow travels through definite pathways in the body called *meridians*. These are associated with the primary organs. Along these 12 meridians lie pressure points which can be pressed or pricked with needles to stimulate the flow of *'chi* and consequently strengthen the relevant organs associated with the illness or problem.

The Chinese relate all the body's functions to five systems, each connected to five internal organs: the liver, the heart, the kidneys, the lungs, and the spleen. The ovaries are actually absent from the picture, whilst the womb is seen as an 'extra organ' whose function is mainly covered by the kidney. Consequently, irregular periods and ovulatory disturbance might be treated with herbs to heal the kidneys. Blocked Fallopian tubes, meanwhile, would be seen to be caused by water retention; as damp and heat are considered related to the liver, yet again it would be the liver that would be treated. The liver is also believed to be responsible for emotional activity, and infertility may be treated as being the result of depression.

There are two main therapies in Chinese medicine: Herbal treatment and acupuncture.

Chinese Herbs

These originate from natural plant, animal and mineral substances. Each has a different nature and function and will be used in combination to promote a therapeutic effect. Herbs are available in different preparations:

Decoctions:	herbs are boiled and the liquid is drunk
Pills:	made of finely ground ingredients absorbed in the body over a long period of time
Granules:	modern formulation based on decoctions mixed with syrup
Extracts:	made by extracting the active ingredients of herbs and then making them into tablets, pills or capsules

Seeing a Chinese Herb Doctor

Much of the success of your treatment will depend on your attitude and the degree of trust you have in the doctor. Normally he or she would see you for an initial consultation lasting up to an hour, during which you might be asked a number of questions about your general health. You might then be prescribed a treatment of herbs, usually taken in cycles of seven days. The herbs are very safe (if sometimes disgusting to taste!), but if you are taking any other drugs prescribed by your GP or fertility specialist you should inform both those doctors and your Chinese Herb doctor about what these are.

Cost

Fees range between £10 and £60 for an initial consultation, plus the cost of the herbs.

Acupuncture

Acupuncture is over 4,500 years old. It is an extremely effective way of rebalancing the body. Acupuncture involves the insertion of small needles just below the skin's surface. It can also involve moxibustion – the burning of herbs over specific points of the body to give warmth. Like herbal medicine, acupuncture works to stimulate our own healing responses, and can promote a general sense of physical and emotional well-being.

In traditional infertility treatment such as IVF, the normal way in which the egg and sperm meet is bypassed. The crucial phase after this is implantation, and a healthy endometrium (womb lining) and internal environment of the uterus are essential. In Chinese medicine the womb needs to be well-nourished by blood and hormones to 'absorb' the yang energy of the sperm. To the acupuncturist, the womb might be 'cold' and the liver function depressed through the woman's own depression or stress. Women with infertility problems usually have menstrual irregularities and may also have pelvic inflammation, vaginal discharge disorders, wasting or obesity problems and, of course, stress, often caused by the infertility problem itself. An acupuncturist would concentrate on regulating the menstrual cycle and strengthening the kidney function. Acupuncture can't always repair internal organs but, as acupuncturist Olivia Wolfe says,

where there is irreversible damage (for example when the Fallopian tubes are damaged) acupuncture attempts to limit the side-effects of IVF technology.

In treating men, the acupuncturist would also concentrate on balancing the energy flow through the system. Research has suggested that acupuncture can have a positive effect on sperm counts and motility.

According to researchers at the University of Heidelburg, Germany, acupuncture may be preferable to hormone treatment. Forty-five infertile women (27 suffering from oligomenorrea and 18 suffering from luteal insufficiency) received a complete gynaecologic-endocrinologic examination before being given a course of treatment with acupuncture. Results were compared to those of 45 women in a control group who received hormone treatment. Both groups were matched for age, duration of infertility, body mass index, previous pregnancies, menstrual cycle and tubal patency ... the acupuncture group had more pregnancies (22/45) than the hormone group (20/45) and none of the women receiving acupuncture suffered from any side-effects. The researchers also observed that the women in the acupuncture group experienced additional health benefits ... and women suffering from various nervous disorders all normalised during the course of acupuncture treatment.

I. GERHARD AND F. POSTNECK, DEPARTMENT OF GYNAECOLOGICAL ENDOCRINOLOGY AND REPRODUCTION, WOMEN'S HOSPITAL, UNIVERSITY OF HEIDELBERG, SEPTEMBER 1992

Seeing an Acupuncturist

Treatment begins with a diagnosis of the energy flow or imbalance. The dysfunction of a *meridian* can be revealed in facial colour, smell, odour, sound of voice, emotional state, taste preference, the patient's symptoms themselves and the distribution of heat and cold on the body.

Fine needles will be applied to different points in the body. The patient is asked to lie still and relax whilst these take an effect. The needles are painless, although some people can feel the electrical charge they can stimulate from the point of insertion along the meridians. Needles will always be sterile, but if you are at all worried about HIV infection you can ask the acupuncturist for reassurance about his or her methods of sterilisation.

Cost

Varies; treatments can last half an hour or one hour. Some practitioners offer a sliding scale of fees. You should expect to pay a minimum of £15 for a shorter session.

There are many thousands of Chinese herbal doctors and acupuncturists working all over the UK. To get a list of fully qualified practitioners in your area, contact The British Acupuncture Council (*see Useful Addresses*).

Homoeopathy

Whilst the roots of homoeopathic medicine can be traced back to the ancient Greeks, the formal system of medicine as we know it today was founded at the end of the 18th century by the German physician Samuel Hahnemann. As with the Chinese medical perspective, in the homoeopathic view the body becomes ill as a result of change in energy patterns or 'vital forces'. Homoeopathy aims to stimulate a person's energy levels. The homoeopath detects imbalances of the organism through subtle symptoms revealed by the individual patient – desire for salt or sugar, sleeping patterns, warmth or coolness of the skin, for example. Therapy consists of matching the vibrational pattern of the symptom with the remedy. This is based on Hahnemann's 'Law of Similars' – 'Like Cures Like'. The word 'homoeopathy' derives from the Greek *homoeo* (similar) and *pathos* (suffering). The idea is that both symptom and cure have a 'personality' and that any substance can either produce or cure illness according to the specific condition (vibrational balance) of the individual receiving it. Each remedy is associated with a specific energy pattern, believed to resonate with the energy pattern of the patient. This resonance of energies between patient and remedy will induce a healing process. Homoeopathic medicines are derived from animals, plants and minerals, concentrated into small pills.

Seeing a Homoeopath

In homoeopathy, as with many 'alternative' practices, the relationship between healer and patient is crucial. The homoeopath isn't a passive observer but engages with the patient to try and 'read' the symptoms.

Cost

Varies, but can be as high as £60 for a consultation.

Massage

There are numerous kinds of massage, all based on the central idea of breaking down tensions in the muscle tissue and promoting a relaxed sense of well-being. Massage is an excellent 'stress-buster' and strongly advised when going through the rigours of infertility treatment and pregnancy itself. In recent years many kinds of massage have been developed or imported from around the world, and masseurs may work with a variety of techniques or a synthesis of their own. The following are two special kinds of massage that may be of special benefit for the infertile person.

Aromatherapy Massage

Aromatherapy is a natural treatment which utilises the therapeutic properties of essential oils, extracted from the flowers, leaves, stems, bark or wood of aromatic plants and trees. It is not a cure-all nor a substitute for medical treatment.
AROMATHERAPIST SUE LEE-TANNER

The medicinal properties of scented flowers, herbs and woods have been known to all the ancient civilisations in Egypt, China, India, Arabia, Greece and Rome. The current revival of interest in 'essential oils' dates back to a man called René Maurice Gattefossé. A chemist in a perfume factory, Gattefossé burned his hand very badly in a laboratory explosion and, on impulse, plunged the injured hand into neat oil of lavender. His hand healed within hours, with no infection. This led to his research into the medicinal uses of lavender and other oils.

Essential oils are extremely potent concentrates. They can be absorbed into the bloodstream via the skin, hair and the lungs (through inhaling). Oils in the bloodstream will circulate for several hours, whilst those inhaled will stimulate the limbic system in the brain, which deals with memory and emotion. It is believed that certain oils will stimulate neurochemicals in the nervous system, but there is as yet insufficient research to prove this.

In massage, tiny amounts of the essential oils would be mixed with other, base oils, such as almond.

Oils of particular relevance to helping with infertility problems are:

Clary Sage: A tonic for the womb and a hormone-balancer. A powerful muscle relaxant which can help with period pains. Has a particularly euphoric and tonic quality, working to promote well-being and energy.

Geranium: Regulates the hormonal system. Can promote vaginal secretion and help with heavy periods. Is also a diuretic, helping poor circulation, and is a tonic to the spirits.

Jasmine: A hormone-balancer and uterine tonic. An anti-depressant and nerve-calming oil. Is said to help men's sperm production. Not to be used in pregnancy, but recommended for childbirth.

Melissa: Regulates menstruation and is a womb tonic. Also a tonic for the heart, calms breathing and uplifts the spirits, soothing the effects of shock and panic.

Rose: A tonic for the womb, it calms PMT, regulates the menstrual cycle and promotes vaginal secretions. Promotes self-confidence and alleviates stress. Is said to increase semen production in men. Can help with sexual difficulties (such as impotence) since it has the power to release the 'happy' hormone dopamine. *NB:* Not to be used in pregnancy.

Ylang Ylang: A hormone-balancer and womb tonic. Is both an anti-depressant and aphrodisiac as well as an antiseptic.

There are of course other beneficial effects from these oils, not least the fact that they smell delicious and, when massaged, you get the added pleasure of hands breaking down your muscular tensions. Besides being massaged into the skin, essential oils can be vaporised by using the oil on a burner or diffuser, inhaled by adding some drops into a bowl of hot water and breathing in the vapours, added to bathwater or, occasionally, applied neat (such as lavender to cuts, stings and burns).

Cost

Varies; minimum £15 upwards.

To find a qualified Aromatherapist, contact the Register of Qualified Aromatherapists (*see Useful Addresses*).

Reflexology

Reflexology is an ancient practice which works along the same principles as acupuncture, but has its own system of energy lines or 'zones'. Reflex points in the feet and hands correspond to parts of the body. Being a biped takes a toll on our feet. When you consider that each foot has 26 bones, 19 muscles and 107 ligaments, and add the full weight which the feet have to support, it isn't surprising that they hold many tensions and blockages. To a reflexologist, the soles of your feet represent a map of your entire body, whilst other features – including skin temperature, texture and puffiness – might indicate internal problems of circulation or glandular imbalances. Applying pressure and massage to the reflexology 'zones' will promote relief from stress, provoke the circulation of energy and encourage the healing process. Your feet feel fantastic afterwards, too!

There are reflex points corresponding to the Fallopian tubes, uterus and prostate, ovary and testes. There are also points which relate to the endocrine system; specific treatment can be given to rebalance reproductive hormone disorders in both men and women.

Going to See a Reflexologist

On initial consultation the practitioner will take a detailed medical history. You will then be asked to sit in a reclining chair or lie down while the reflexologist examines your feet. The massage is mainly applied by the thumb. Pressure is used and there may be parts of the foot which are exceptionally sensitive. Whilst this may be slightly painful, it is the kind of deep releasing pain (experienced in, for example, back massage when your shoulders are tense) and hence ultimately pleasurable!

Cost

Varies; you should expect to pay £25 and upwards for one hour's treatment.

Hypnotherapy

Hypnotherapy basically works on the subconscious via guided relaxation and visualisation techniques. Since stress is proven to affect menstrual cycles and sperm production, to an extent it would be true to say that fertility in some cases is actually controlled by our subconscious and that it might therefore be guided towards positive results. Some hypnotherapists even believe that a condition such as spasmodically blocked tubes (ie where there is no impairment causing the tubes to close) can be cured as can sperm concentration, count and motility.

Seeing a Hypnotherapist

The experience of hypnotherapy is of being encouraged into a state of deep relaxation. From this the therapeutic process proceeds via suggestion. A hypnotherapist discusses the history of infertility with the patient. Hypnosis is then gradually induced by talking gently about the reproductive system and its processes, asking the patient to visualise this in detail. All the while the hypnotherapist encourages the patient to feel positive about themselves and about the possibility of becoming pregnant. During this process of positive thinking s/he might ask questions about anything in the patient's past which might be impeding a pregnancy from occurring, always being sure to re-enforce the idea of success and of eliminating fears. The Hypnotherapy Association (see addresses) works on a long term basis with the patient and its hypnotherapists are trained psychotherapists, as opposed to the school of simple suggestion hypnotherapy which might involve a one-off session only.

Cost

Varies. You should expect to pay well over £40 for a 50 minute session to see a specialist via the Hypnotherapy Association.

DIY Stress-busting

If you find the point of balance (rest)
in the body,
You can easily settle the details.
If you settle the details,
You will stop rushing around.
If you stop rushing around,
Your mind will become calm.
If your mind becomes calm,
You can think in front of a Tiger.
If you can think in front of a Tiger,
You will surely succeed.
MENCIUS (ANCIENT CHINESE PHILOSOPHER)

We now know that stress is bad for the health, and research continues to locate exactly why stress has a deleterious effect on fertility. Normal levels of stress associated with the failure to conceive are only compounded by tests, investigations and treatment itself. There are many ways to stress-bust. One obvious way is to look at your lifestyle and check out what you are actually doing every day. You might be someone who has overworked for years, possibly to (unconsciously) numb the pain of childlessness. You may have a busy career in a competitive environment and feel that you have to put in long hours with no lunchbreaks or proper holidays to hold your position in the field. You may be in a job which is simply stressful in itself. The list is endless.

The coordinator of the clinic I attended reminded me recently how I had arrived for my first IVF appointments with a bulging Filofax, in a highly stressful job and feeling extra hassled by how I would 'fit it all in' and manage the treatment cycle without interrupting my work commitments. I soon learnt! If you are involuntarily infertile you owe it to yourself to try and alter your stressful lifestyle to help you get through your treatment. If a baby is the happy result, your lifestyle will change anyway (as will the sources of stress), so you may as well start now.

The most natural way to stress-bust is to get enough sleep. The second is to exercise regularly. You may loathe the idea of sweating and straining at the local aerobics class. There are far more simple and healthy ways of getting your muscles stretched and your blood circulating. Walking is an obvious one. Other forms of exercise which are quiet and can (once learnt) be practised at home are Yoga and T'ai 'Chi.

Yoga

This ancient Indian movement art involves exercises to stretch the muscles and joints and control the breath. Soft versions of yoga exercises are now used by many antenatal teachers, particularly those specialising in Active Birth antenatal classes.

T'ai 'Chi

This is an ancient Chinese 'soft' martial-art. Its principles relate to those of Chinese medicine and acupuncture. The circulation of *'chi* energy in the body and the constant flow between states of *yin* and *yang* are central. A sequence of movements is studied and practised daily, promoting a relaxed mind and coordinated body.

Meditation

There are many systems of meditation, mainly from India, Tibet, China and Japan. Meditation involves relaxing the mind by concentrating on a *mantra* (sound pattern) or light (flame) or on the movement of your own breath. Meditation usually involves sitting still in a certain posture and 'observing' your breath, then controlling it. Meditation is normally taught in groups and practised on a daily basis at home. Its ultimate aim is for spiritual enlightenment. Along the way it can promote a calmer and less anxious response mechanism to the stresses of daily life, and counteracts depression.

Diet (We Are What We Eat...)

Whilst you may envy the teenage mum on the High Street eating a bag of crisps and smoking a cigarette, poor diet not only affects our health but is proven to affect fertility and reduce the health or life-expectancy of a child. A balanced diet is essential to promote general health, but is particularly advised when trying to get pregnant. Not only will your own bodies (I'm talking of the couple here!) be fitter and stronger, but the woman will be preparing herself in a positive way for carrying a baby to term. Being nourished in the womb is the most crucial time in a baby's development.

A balanced diet should include carbohydrates, fats, proteins, vitamins, minerals and roughage. You should try and avoid junk food (full of chemical additives) and over-refined carbohydrates (white sugar and flour). Cut down on animal fats and try and eat your proteins as fresh as possible. The fresher your food, the higher its vitamin and mineral content, since over-cooking and processing can kill these essential nutrients. Calcium – found in dairy products, fish, nuts and dried fruit – is essential to build healthy teeth and bones and important in preventing pregnancy-induced pre-eclampsia (hypertension) and calcium depletion leading to osteoporosis in later life. Iron, essential for the development of your blood supply, isn't only found in spinach but in sardines, jacket potatoes, certain pulses (chick peas, lentils, kidney beans), dried fruits and soya products. Vitamin C is found in many fruits and vegetables such as citrus fruits, tomatoes, broccoli, cauliflower and cabbage. It is essential for tissue repair and can boost your resistance to infections such as colds and flu. Roughage is the fibre in food which keeps the digestive tract functioning, and is thought to help prevent intestinal cancer. If you try and eat as much unrefined grain and fresh fruit and vegetables as possible you will get your daily supply and keep 'regular'. Whilst this may not have any direct influence on your fertility, constipation can be painful, uncomfortable and leave you feeling sluggish and depressed. Caffeine, found in tea and some soft drinks like coca-cola as well as coffee, is actually an 'addictive' substance. Research suggests that it has a bad effect on sperm motility (causing immobilisation in large amounts) and can cause miscarriage and foetal abnormalities. Alcohol, like smoking, is known to depress sperm motility and function (as well as a man's capacity for erection) and can affect foetal development.

Tips for Healthy Eating
- Buy organic if available and affordable.
- Eat fresh rather than frozen or tinned.
- Eat plenty of raw fruit and vegetables.
- Steam rather than boil.
- 'Stir fry', grill, roast or stew rather than deep fry.
- Avoid re-heated meals and try and eat as soon after preparation as possible.
- Reduce animal fats.
- Drink plenty of mineral or filtered water.
- Cut down on alcohol.
- Cut down on caffeine.

- Cut down on refined carbohydrates.
- Eat fibre-rich foods.
- Take a daily vitamin and mineral supplement.

Why All the Effort on Top of Everything Else?

Thinking about a sensible, balanced diet and setting yourself some light fitness and stress-busting programme can be a really positive way of taking control of your own body. It shouldn't feel like an added pressure but a way of preparing yourself mentally and physically for the challenge of treatment. If you are low in energy and unfit, you will be more easily depressed by obstacles. If you are fit and in a positive frame of mind and spirit, you will be able to cope better and remain in control of a process which can all too often feel high-tech, oppressive and alienating. Furthermore, your general health will be taken into account by the clinic. If you are generally fit and well and free of addictions you stand a much better chance of a speedy recovery following any operations or treatment cycles. To certain doctors your general health and fitness may well determine how seriously you are taken as a prospective patient, or how soon after a failed IVF cycle you will be advised to try again.

A specialist organisation which can help you get fit for pregnancy, and increase the odds all round is called Foresight.

Foresight

A major shift needs to take place from the assumption that a substance is safe until it is proven otherwise, to the position that it is dangerous until proven safe!
BELINDA BARNES AND SUZANNE GAIL BRADLEY, *PLANNING FOR A HEALTHY BABY*
(VERMILION, 1994)

Foresight – The Association for The Promotion of Preconceptual Care – was founded in 1978 with a mission to pioneer preconceptual care through nutritional medicine. Its dual objective is to safeguard the health of the unborn child through preconceptual care and to promote the study of the effects of the environment on preconceptual care. Vigilant in its research and thorough in its treatment, Foresight aims to prepare men's and women's bodies at least six months before conceiving a baby, so that uterus, ova and sperm are all in tip-top condition. Counteracting pollutants of the modern world – smoking, alcohol, pesticides, food additives, lead and toxic metals – and the resulting vitamin and mineral deficiencies are at the centre of its work. A whole range of infertility causes have been traced back to vitamin and mineral deficiencies or the presence of toxic metals in the body. Dietary factors and allergies have also been proven to play their part. Certain essential nutrients, even if eaten, might not be being absorbed in the body (malabsorption) due to the presence of Candida albicans in the gut. This is a yeast-like organism normally experienced as 'thrush' in the genital area or sometimes the mouth. It can take on a fungal form and penetrate the gut wall. Current research suggests that there may well be a link between infertility in women and Candida albicans, and that cutting down on sugar and alcohol (which promote the growth of this yeast) can help. This is just one of the many fascinating areas of knowledge which mainstream medicine often misses and which Foresight will help locate and treat.

Once you have been diagnosed, treatment will involve a controlled allergy-free diet plan and vitamin and mineral supplements to detoxify the body of any traces of elements which might be preventing you from achieving a healthy pregnancy. Whilst Foresight practitioners don't claim to cure structural problems such as blocked Fallopian tubes (although studies suggest that low magnesium levels can impede tubal muscular action), they have achieved remarkable results, notably in older women, cases of poor sperm counts and 'unexplained' infertility. Their overall success rate is 86 per cent, whilst their success rate for IVF in conjunction with the Foresight method is 65 per cent. These astonishing results do not affect just subfertility itself. The overall health of the babies born is significant, with high birthweights and reduced birth abnormalities. Foresight is especially advised for cases of 'unexplained' or 'secondary' infertility, though there is no reason why, even with a tubal diagnosis and planned IVF treatment, you shouldn't use the Foresight method as a complementary approach. Foresight Founder Belinda Barnes argues that ART methods such as ICSI are unnecessary since poor sperm production can be treated through nutritional methods and vitamin and mineral control. She recommends that any couple contemplating IVF should contact Foresight first, since some clinics may advise IVF when in fact this extreme course of action may not be necessary. She also advocates 'natural' IVF – that is, without superovulation hormone drugs.

Foresight produce a pocketbook on food additives, *Find Out*, and a cookbook, *The Foresight Wholefood Cookbook*, as well as several pamphlets explaining the adverse effects of harmful substances, from smoking to lead, in detail. They also produce the book *Planning for a Healthy Baby* and the video *Preparing for the Healthier Baby*. When you join you also will be given a list of local organic food suppliers, although these days it is common to find organic produce in the big supermarkets.

THE BASIC FORESIGHT PLAN

Six months prior to intended conception both partners should:

- Eat a wholefood diet, free from dangerous additives and organically produced where possible.
- Use natural family planning.
- Have mineral analyses done, and follow the programmes of supplementation and cleansing to rid the body of toxic metals and to balance levels of essential minerals as indicated. Retest as advised.
- Filter all water used in drinking and cooking with a Kenwood or Boots Crystal Water Filter.
- Check with your dentist that (s)he isn't still using mercury amalgams.
- Have tests for Rubella status, toxoplasmosis, allergies, thyroid function, enzyme functioning, chlamydia, genital bacteria infections, malabsorption and Candida albicans. Have any immunisation, treatment or adapted diet as advised. *NB:* Dietary manipulation can clear up most allergies without drugs.
- Both partners should test for genito-urinary infection. Immediately treat any infection present.
- Eliminate smoking, alcohol and all but the absolutely necessary drugs prescribed by your GP (and check if they are contraindicated in pregnancy).
- Avoid the use of organophosphate pesticides in the home, or any food or materials treated with pesticides.
- Check with your dentist that (s)he isn't still using mercury amalgams.

How to Join Foresight

Send an SAE with a 33p stamp (*see Useful Addresses*).

You will then be sent the address of your Branch Secretary and information about local Foresight clinicians and nutritionists. The clinician will be a qualified doctor. You will be given information about the Foresight principles and the address of your local Natural Family Planning teacher.

Costs

Joining Foresight costs £17.63 per annum. Your Foresight clinician may charge anything from £40 to £100 for a consultation. The cost of vitamins and mineral supplements will vary according to your prescription.

And last, but not least, a word about:

Magic and Superstition

You wouldn't be the first infertile person to practise some kind of magic or become highly superstitious. This might be about your menstruation, your treatment or any resulting pregnancy. People have practised fertility cults since prehistoric times, using herbs, potions, prayer, imagery, icons and ritual. You may find yourself naturally drawn to finding your own rituals or reading your own signs into things around you. You may find yourself creating taboos around certain objects, foodstuffs or even people you suspect interfere with your well-being and the success of your treatment. This doesn't mean you are losing your reason and it is nothing to be ashamed about. It is a normal and natural consequence of the powerlessness you feel about your fertility, and the stress and strain you are going through. Your own personal 'voodoo' may be your unconscious way of protecting yourself against things (and people) which add to your stress in some way. We don't all have our Angel Gabriels to give us good news, and many of us may not belong to a church nor have a faith to guide us. Without these 'props' to lean on, it is very human to find that the profound experience of infertility awakens deep spiritual needs, a search for higher meanings and a desperate longing for comfort in the midst of a high-tech and seemingly soul-less process.

1. Actually in medicine intuition plays a part in the clinician's practice and there is an increasing acknowledgement that the mind might play a part in the healing process. Infertility doctors, for instance, generally accept the view that stress may affect fertility, and research continues to try and discover how and why.

CHAPTER (6)

Adoption and Fostering

① Adoption

Son: (angrily) 'You're not my real mother!'
Mother: 'Yes I am, I wash your underpants!'

The mother in this scene was Jacqueline Paschoud, Chair of the ACU Patient Support Group at King's College Hospital in London. She told it to an audience at the 'Angels and Mechanics' Conference in London in June 1996, to illustrate her point that as a mother of one 'spontaneous' child, two children who were adopted and one born through IVF, parenting is a job as much as a biological destiny. You mother because you nurture. Involuntarily childless people invariably seek the production of their own genetic child as a first choice. Adoption and fostering tend to get put on the bottom of the list of preferred options. Certainly the biological drive to reproduce can be ferocious, but any parent of children who have been adopted will tell you that the love and bonding they feel for the child(ren) is as powerful as that they feel for any genetically linked one.

The gradual changes in society as regards gender roles and sexual choice are helping to show us that there is an important distinction between wanting to have a baby and wanting to parent. The desire for a family, over and above any desire by a woman to be pregnant and give birth, is the enduring reality of parenthood. Pregnancy is an extraordinarily powerful experience and childbirth a rite of passage for women, but once those little feet patter in your home (whatever their origins) you are legally, practically and emotionally responsible for their owners: You are a parent.

Adoption really does put 'the welfare of the child' issue at the centre of attention. Whilst your own needs for a child are obviously respected, adoption agencies will concentrate not on what the child can offer you but on what you can offer the child. Furthermore, unlike having a baby of your own, there is no statutory maternity leave for adoption. All the research involved, your applications, 'homestudy' (by the social worker) and, in the case of overseas adoption, any necessary travel abroad (and finance for this) will come out of your own time and be your own responsibility.

There are black babies waiting for black families and babies with disabilities who need new homes. But if you are white and have set your heart on adopting a healthy white baby you should be prepared for a long wait; and you should accept that you may eventually be disappointed as very few such children need adoption.

ABOUT ADOPTION AND FOSTERING, BRITISH AGENCIES FOR ADOPTION AND FOSTERING PAMPHLET

When people think of adopting they immediately dream of a little baby they can nurture from infancy and on whom they can lavish all their love and cuddles, someone they can watch take the first steps or speak a first word.

Actually, in the UK very few small babies are available for adoption thanks to the wider availability of contraception and abortion, more lenient attitudes and State income support to young unmarried mothers. For example, in England and Wales the number of babies under one year old who were adopted dropped from 2,945 in 1977 to 895 in 1991, and in Scotland from 291 in 1983 to 71 in 1992.[1]

Today the greatest need for adoption is among older children and children with physical or learning impairments. Some of these children will have behavioural problems associated with experiences of abuse or family insecurity. Among them may be groups of siblings who don't want to be separated but adopted as a unit. Agencies may refer to all these cases as children with 'special needs' as a way of alerting you to the challenging job which may lie ahead if you adopt them, and the kind of stamina and commitment you may need in order to cope. On top of all this, most agencies will only place healthy babies with parents who are married and aged between 21 and 35 (40 for the man). Because of the surplus of children with special needs, these rules will become far more flexible in these cases. Your financial situation will be taken into account to ensure that you can afford to bring up the child(ren); you may be paid an Adoption Allowance to help with costs.

Adoption is a legal procedure. When you adopt you take on full parental responsibility for the child(ren) you adopt. Until now, some people have found the realities of adopting in the UK testing to the point of deterrence. They might have exceeded the age limit, not conform to lifestyle regulations, or have set their heart on adopting a young baby. Many such people have decided to look overseas to poorer countries which sadly yield up many more unwanted babies than we do. Political events and media attention produce trends – Romania following the removal of Ceaucescu when the plight of children in orphanages was revealed, for example, or the People's Republic of China following the highly emotive TV Documentary *The Dying Rooms*.

Adoption facts:

58,000 children are in local authority care
5,000 are suitable for adoption
Only 50 per cent get matched to a family
There are currently 1,300 couples waiting to adopt

Tony Blair's government has recognised the adoption procedures both in the UK and for overseas adoption need modernisation in the interests of 'the needs and rights of the child at the centre of the process' (Executive Summary, Performance and Innovation Unit report on adoption 2000). In 1999 The Inter-Country Aspects Adoption Act was passed and will be implemented in 2001. The Department of Health is in the process of writing the guidelines for this which will be published in the spring of 2001 (for any enquiries, or to obtain copies of this report please consult the Department of Health , see the Addresses section at the back of the book). Blair commissioned The Performance and Innovation Report of July 2000 to conduct a study and make recommendations to the government (available on the web – see Addresses section at the back of the book). To give some idea of Blair's message of commitment to adopters and adoptees, here is what he states in the foreword to the PIU Report:

I am determined to make early progress. It is clear from the PIU report that there are some things we can get on with quickly. Over the next few months we will therefore:

- *Develop and implement proposals for a National Adoption Register, to co-ordinate those waiting to adopt with children needing new families, and so cut out unnecessary delays.*
- *Draw up a new National Standards, which Local Authorities will need to follow, setting out timescales for making decisions about children and clear criteria for assessing adopters, so that children do not drift in care and those wanting to adopt know what to expect and can be confident they will be treated fairly;*
- *Set up an Adoption and Permanency Taskforce, to spread best practice, tackle poor performance and to help all Local Authorities reach the standards of the best;*
- *Conduct a rapid scrutiny of the backlog of children waiting to be placed with adoptive families and approved adopters waiting for children, to see if any suitable matches can be made*

The Government is committed to modernising adoption.

On 21st December 2000 a government White Paper was published in which the Health Secretary Alan Milburn said he aimed to increase the annual rate of adoption by 40 per cent by the year 2005. Key issues covered in the White Paper include: the placement of children in mixed race couples, eliminating blanket bans on prospective parents because of age, health or other factors, speeding up the whole process (which currently takes around 3 years) and pledging:

Proper financial support for families who have adopted together with good post-adoption support ... Adoption is not a cheap option so these changes will require extra money from the government to local authorities to ensure they happen.

As for adopting from overseas, whilst certain legal requirements such as homestudies will now conform to UK adoption regulations, there will continue to be specific factors to consider before embarking on such a route. Time, commitment and cost are just two of the crucial factors here. In situ research in the country from which you wish to adopt is essential as you will need to make an educated and informed choice, in addition to the obligatory visit of both parties (where a couple is involved) to fetch the child. Agencies abroad and legal costs can amount to thousands of pounds.

The cases of couples adopting abroad and getting into trouble are well documented. The media really enjoyed the scandal involving the imprisonment of adopters in Romania.

They love to produce articles about illegal adoptions, baby buying, baby selling, baby stealing etc. THERE IS NO NEED TO GET INVOLVED IN ANY OF THESE PRACTICES.

Adoptions can be done legally, safely and absolutely free of charge from many countries. Several countries have established a framework to facilitate the adoption of orphaned and abandoned children by suitable people from other countries. Even in countries where an established system is not operating, adoptions can often be arranged by reputable lawyers or registered adoption agencies.

OASIS: GENERAL GUIDE TO OVERSEAS ADOPTION, 1996

There are so many examples of the happiness and fulfilment brought to adopters and their children from abroad that it isn't my place to sermonise here at all. In so many cases adopting such children might be giving them a far brighter future than the one they could expect remaining in orphanages in their home country. However, it is worth considering a caveat in CHILD's factsheet on adoption:

Many poorer countries may need help in caring for some of their children, but adoption is not usually the best way of achieving this. Taking a child away from its country of origin should only be considered if there is no realistic prospect of that child being adopted in its own country. There may be fewer babies for adoption in this country, but there are hundreds of other children in this country that you can offer a home to, before considering overseas adoption.

Clearly this is the message of the Government's reforms also, namely to encourage more prospective adopters in the UK by creating a speedier, more attractive and user-friendly social, legal and economic environment in which this option might supersede all others. But each individual or couple will have different responses here and that is why if you are thinking of adopting you should first research your opportunities and choices thoroughly. Useful first-stop organisations include the British Agencies for Adoption and Fostering (BAAF), the Parent to Parent Information on Adoption Services (PPIAS) and the Overseas Adoption Helpline. You might also contact voluntary support groups for overseas adoption such as OASIS or the post-adoption Guatemalan Families Association (which accepts pre-adopters into their group) to get advice from those who have direct hands-on experience. You are also advised to contact your Local Authority Social Services Department (who will put you in touch with adoption agencies – there are nearly 200 of these currently in the UK), the Department of Health and Home Office Immigration. All of these addresses (apart from your Local Authority) can be found in the Addresses section at the back of this book.

British Agencies for Adoption and Fostering (BAAF)

BAAF is a professional association for people and organisations working in the field of childcare or who are involved with adoption and fostering. Its members include almost all Local Authority and voluntary adoption agencies in Scotland, England and Wales, plus associate members and a list of 1,500 individual members including childcare and allied professionals.
   BAAF's mission is to:

- promote and develop high standards in adoption and fostering for childcare and other professionals
- promote public understanding of adoption and fostering, and raise awareness of the special circumstances, including the racial, cultural, religious and linguistic needs of children and young people separated from their birth families
- act as an independent voice in the field of childcare, to inform and influence policy-makers and legislators, and all those responsible for the welfare of children and young people
- work within a child-centred, multi-disciplinary and anti-discriminatory framework, working with all statutory agencies and voluntary organisations concerned with childcare but with a focus on fostering and adoption.

BAAF, working in the best interests of children and young people, implements this mission by influencing policy and practice at a governmental, professional and media level by providing training and consultancy, finding families for children, offering a public advice and information service and producing a wide range of books, pamphlets and periodicals (a journal and a family-finding newspaper) for the public, as well as professional literature. BAAF also has specialist groups operating both regionally and nationally – legal and medical groups, for example, and the Black Perspectives Advisory Committee.

Overseas Adoption Helpline

OAH is an information and advice service providing:

- written information and telephone advice concerning inter-country adoption requirements and procedures in the UK, including the Overseas Adoption Helpline Procedural Guide to Intercountry Adoption
- written information on the adoption requirements and procedures of other countries which place children for inter-country adoption, including factsheets about the requirements and procedures in various countries
- in a majority of cases, details of the services to prospective inter-country adopters which are available in their local area. These include a named person to contact, the fees charged for carrying out a homestudy, and the time-scales involved.

To contact these and other organisations please see the Useful Addresses chapter (*page 276*).

Positive Adoption Language

Positive Adoption Language (PAL) is based on the ideas of Marietta Spencer, an adoption social worker who has been evolving the ideas of PAL for 20 years.[II]

PAL is a vocabulary relating to adoption which bestows respect, dignity, responsibility and objectivity to the decisions made by birth and adoptive parents. It is designed to eliminate the societally-held myth that adoption is the 'second best' to form a family and that by being involved in adoption one has actually missed out on a 'real' family experience.

Through adoption, parent and child are linked by love and law. The fact that they are not connected by blood has often meant that some people are unwilling to acknowledge the relationship as genuine and permanent. So they use qualifiers ('This is Bill's adopted son') in situations where they would not dream of doing so in a non-adoptive family ('This is Bill's birth-control-failure son' or 'This is Mary's Caesarean-section daughter').

Some people don't assign a full and permanent relationship to persons related through adoption ('Do you have children of your own?' or 'Have you met the natural mother?' or 'Are they real brothers and sisters?'). They assume adoptive relationships are tentative ('Can you give her back if she has medical problems?').

The reality is that adoption is a method of joining a family, just as is birth. Adoption should never be thought of as a 'condition'. In most articles or situations not centring on adoption, it is inappropriate to mention adoption. (The exception is of course an arrival announcement).

When it is appropriate to mention adoption, it is correct to say 'Kathy was adopted' (referring to the way in which she arrived in her family in the past tense). Phrasing it in the present tense implies that adoption is a condition that colours all facets of one's life. After all, with a birth child we say 'Kathy was born on the 2nd of April.'

Those who raise and nurture a child are his parents. In describing family relationships involving adoption, it is best to avoid terms such as 'real' or 'natural'. Also, one should never refer to a birth-child as 'one of my own'. This intimates that genetic relationships are stronger and more enduring than adoptive relationships.

The process by which families prepare themselves to become parents is often called a homestudy. This term carries with it the old view of the process as a weeding out or judgement. More and more adoption authorities are beginning to view their roles as less God-like and more facilitative. The preferred, positive term is 'parent preparation'.

For children born outside the United Kingdom, we should use the term international adoption. The older term 'foreign' has negative connotations in other uses ('the whole idea is foreign to me' or 'I don't like it, it seems so foreign').

QUOTED IN 'MOSAIC' – THE OASIS NEWSLETTER. AUTUMN 1995.

Telling a Child about His or Her Origins

In the old days before children's needs were fully understood, information about adopted children's birth parents tended to be buried and suppressed. It is now generally recognised that, however happy people may have been to be brought up by their adoptive parents, they will reach a point in their lives when they may desperately want to know their origins. Adoption agencies encourage adoptive parents to talk to the child(ren) at appropriate moments in their development and tell them how they came to be adopted and, possibly, facts about their parental background. As adoptive parents, your child(ren)'s questions may naturally make you feel insecure. Adoption agencies would encourage people to come to them for advice and counselling if information-giving is proving painful or a source of conflict or trauma in the family.

The Adoption Act of 1976 (amended by the Children Act of 1989) gave adoptees in England and Wales the right to see their birth certificates and know more about their origins at the age of 18. In Scotland the age is 17. Many adults who were adopted use this information to search for their birth parents. People who were born prior to the Children Act was passed and who want access to their birth records have to have a meeting with a counsellor at their Social Services Department or at the voluntary agency which arranged their adoption. People born after this date can choose whether to see a counsellor or not. The Children Act also means that, in theory, birth parents can ask the court to let them apply for contact with their child(ren).

ⓘ Fostering

On a day-to-day parenting basis, fostering is no different from adoption. You take care of the child's needs, emotional, medical, social and educational. If you already have children, you integrate the fostered child(ren) into your family as one of your own. The difference is that when you foster a child or children you don't become their legal parents and usually share the care of the child(ren) with their birth parents. For this reason the National Foster Care Association prefer to use the term 'foster carer' for the person(s) fostering the child(ren). The birth parents may visit you regularly or the child(ren) may go and stay with them. Children who need fostering are those who for whatever reason are vulnerable in their home situation. The family unit may have broken down in some way, or the child may have behavioural problems or a disability. Whatever the reason, the birth parents are in crisis and can't cope on their own and the child(ren) will probably be suffering as a result. The Local Authority takes such children into their care and social workers are appointed to the case. They will endeavour to help the family sort out their problems and they will develop strategies for the child(ren)'s future both in the short and long term.

The couple or family who foster a child(ren) may only have them for a short period of time. Sometimes, however, the foster child(ren) might wish to remain with their foster family on a permanent basis while still retaining their legal ties with their birth parents. In certain adoption cases, prospective parents may be required to foster the child for a period of adjustment so that both parties can get used to each other before the full commitment of adoption.

Foster carers receive an allowance to cover costs, which may vary from area to area. Depending on the agency and the type of fostering you do, you may also be paid a (taxable) fee.

The social worker(s) will retain a relationship with the child and carers, perhaps taking the child on outings and responding to any arising needs. Foster parents will also be regularly checked by their social worker.

The interval between applying to foster and being approved can be long since a lot of bureaucracy is involved. Prospective foster carers will undergo an assessment by social workers. This homestudy, as with adoption, will include a check on your records and will endeavour to find out about you and your home life through meetings with a social worker in your own home. You would also have a short period of training because it is likely that the child(ren) you foster will be confused and troubled. They will have undergone a major upheaval in their lives and may have mild to severe behavioural difficulties.

Looking after children has become an increasingly complex and risky business for foster carers. The majority of children placed today have more difficult and disturbed patterns of behaviour than they did twenty years ago.
NATIONAL FOSTER CARE ASSOCIATION REPORT

As a carer you may find it frustrating that whilst you have the day-to-day care of the child(ren) you have few legal rights and no parental responsibility. Being with the child(ren) 24 hours a day means you'll feel you understand their needs better than anyone, yet the agency might have different views from you. Inevitably disputes and differences may arise between the carers and agencies.

They make so many mistakes ... two years ago when he was having problems (he'd been expelled from school) they wanted him to go to boarding school. We disagreed with that. We said it would make it worse. It would make him feel rejected a second time. Anyway, he didn't want to go. We said 'no' and stuck to our guns all the way and in the end they said we'd made the right decision.
FOSTER PARENTS OF A BOY, NOW 14, WHO HAS LIVED WITH THEM SINCE HE WAS
2 YEARS OLD

Foster carers can feel powerless. Problems may arise with the child(ren)'s family, they may feel isolated and may also be vulnerable to allegations of abuse since they are often caring for children who are emotionally damaged. As a foster carer you may treat the child(ren) you foster as your own, but in the end if you know the child(ren) will soon be returning to their birth parents you'll probably find a need to hold back from becoming too attached. So all in all, fostering demands great strength of mind, stability and compassion.

The NFCA Advice and Mediation Service

The National Foster Care Association established an Advice and Mediation Service in 1989 to respond to the stress foster carers can experience. This service was set up to:

- offer advice and support to foster carers where an independent source of help is appropriate, for example allegations of abuse from carers, proposed terminations of approval, and complaints by carers about agency decisions
- mediate between carers and agencies when invited to do so
- contribute to agency policies, procedures and training programmes which promote 'safe caring' practices and help keep allegations and complaints to a minimum.

In April 1994 they set up an Advice Line dealing with all kinds of enquiries and needs for support by carers. You can join the NFCA and as a member receive a quarterly magazine, discounts on training schemes, a range of free publications and a 24-hour legal advice service and legal costs insurance. To contact the NFCA, see the Useful Addresses chapter (*page 276*).

Fostering can and will be exhausting and sometimes your patience will be stretched to the limit. But the rewards are there as well: the satisfaction of seeing the child and parents happily reunited, a sense of breakthrough when a young person finally starts to talk to you, the delights when an unhappy toddler smiles. Foster children aren't like your own children and love is not enough to enable you to look after them ... In caring for children you will be fostering not only them, but their families, their past, their future. There are few tasks that could be more important to the well-being of children and the wider community.

CARING AND SHARING IS FOSTERING (NFCA PUBLICATION 1001)

If you are interested in becoming a foster carer, you should contact your Local Authority Social Services or Social Work Department.

CHAPTER ⑦

The Body Politic

Science, by itself, cannot supply us with an ethic.
BERTRAND RUSSELL

① The Human Fertilisation and Embryology Authority

It is an extremely rare thing: a quango with democratic principles. It is powerful. Those who contravene the law it patrols and its codes risk prison. It is tied up with rules that forbid disclosures because of the sensitivity of its work. It deals with some of the most controversial issues of our time. Yet the HFEA could not be less controversial or less adversarial, or more willing to seek and accept the views of lay people. And then to act on them.
THE INDEPENDENT, 7TH JANUARY 1994

Louise Brown, born in the UK in 1978, was the world's first 'test-tube' baby and heralded nothing short of a reproductive revolution. Debates in Parliament and the media in the wake of her birth were rife. The Committee of Inquiry into Human Fertilisation and Embryology, led by Mary Warnock, was consequently set up. What then became known as the 'Warnock Report' recommended to Parliament and the House of Lords that a statutory body should be elected to monitor the rapid technological advances in reproductive medicine. What immediately followed was the creation of the Voluntary (later Interim) Licencing Authority for Human In Vitro Fertilisation and Embryology (ILA) in 1985. This self-regulating body continued operating until 1990, when the Human Fertilisation and Embryology Act was passed in Parliament. This Act required the convening of a national regulatory body – the Human Fertilisation and Embryology Authority (HFEA) – an independent organisation established by Parliament in 1991 and funded by a combination of license fees from clinics (per treatment cycle) and a Government Grant.

The HFEA is a quango. Its 19 members, plus Chairman and Deputy, are appointed by the State. Under new Government procedures following the guidelines of the Nolan Report, 'Standards in Public Life', a few fresh members are recruited each year, vacancies are advertised and appointments made by interview. Members work with a team of Inspectors to oversee the licensing and good practice of all UK clinics both in the NHS and the private sector. Their main role is to monitor IVF, DI, embryo research and cryopreservation. The HFEA remit is ethical, legal, social and medical. Under the law its other functions include:

- keeping a formal register of information about donors, treatments and children born from those treatments so that children born from donor gametes can have access to certain facts about their genetic history
- producing a Code of Practice giving guidelines to clinics about the proper conduct of licensed activities
- publicising its role and providing information to patients, donors and clinics
- keeping 'under review' information about embryos, the development of those embryos and the provision of treatment services and activities governed by the HF & E Act.

The HFEA makes recommendations to Parliament based on its internal debates. It has also, as in the case of the possible use of ovarian tissue from aborted foetuses, opened up debate to the public by publishing reports and inviting comment.

> At least half the HFEA members are not doctors or scientists involved in research or practice relevant to infertility.[1]

As a public body, HFEA is keenly user-friendly. It produces public information leaflets about treatments, consultative documents about certain issues, and an annual Patient's Guide to Licensed Clinics. It can get up the infertility experts' nose because it interferes with their freedom, demands reams of paperwork on a regular basis, and sometimes threatens to or actually removes a licence. Consultants may grumble about 'the nanny state', but actually as a fertility treatment 'consumer' you may be reassured to know that a group of 20 or so people are constantly checking that work in the field is conducted in an ethical and proper fashion.

Is the HFEA Necessary?

Professor Robert Winston did recently claim that the science of ART was
actually slowing down and that 'the world is safe from me.'[1] But all kinds
of genetic research is going on in the world's laboratories, with enormous
moral and ethical implications. Also, occasional but disturbing cases of
unethical practice on the part of ART consultants have come to light, such
as the doctor who cheated on declaring the amount of eggs and embryos he
was acquiring from patients so as to boost his bank of gametes, and a case
in the US of a doctor who was jailed for being discovered to have been using
his own sperm exclusively in treating patients who needed donor sperm.
Obviously these incidents are exceptions. However, let's not forget that the
medical profession is extremely hierarchical, patriarchal and competitive,
and that fertility treatment has turned the previously lacklustre specialism
of obstetrics and gynaecology into a sexy, virile and high-tech branch of
medicine. Power corrupts. And what could be more powerful than having
the technology to create life itself? So, arguably, without such a restraining
body as the HFEA some of the excesses of which we are rightly afraid might
indeed have become widespread.

The Daily Express reported in May 1996 that, at the University of
Pennsylvania in the US, a biologist had engineered a mouse which
produced rat sperm by implanting the stem cells from the rat into the
mouse's testes. The logical conclusion of this research is that it may be
possible in the future for one man to produce the sperm of another,
introducing for the first time the concept of surrogate fatherhood.

As laypeople we continue to be astounded by what a bit of tinkering in the
infertility lab might be capable of producing. The reality of genetic
engineering is with us, not to mention certain techniques which we find
abhorrent (what's known in the trade as a 'yuk factor'). For most of us it is
hard to imagine scientists restraining themselves from the temptation to
stray further and further away from the hands-on and rather commonplace
job of helping a couple conceive into the realms of super-high-tech
manipulations of Nature. Breaking boundaries goes with the job. So
whatever irritant to free practice such a body might be, in principle at least
it is certainly in the interests of the infertile public. It follows that it is

therefore vital that the HFEA itself remains a democratic body, that members are selected to represent the widest cross-section of the British public, and that it keeps in touch with the general public's views and feelings on the subject.

Of one thing, I have no doubt. The growing use of reprogenetics is inevitable. For better and *worse, a new age is upon us – an age in which we as humans will gain the ability* to change the nature of our species.

LEE M. SILVER: *REMAKING EDEN – HOW GENETIC ENGINEERING AND CLONING WILL TRANSFORM THE AMERICAN FAMILY*, AVON BOOKS, NEW YORK 1997, ISBN: 0 380 79243 5.

ⓘⓘ Issues

It is not, as the bio-moralists claim, that scientific innovation has outstripped our social and moral codes. Just the opposite is the case. Their obsession with the life of the embryo has deflected our attention away from the real issue, which is how the babies that are born are raised and nurtured. The ills in our society have nothing to do with assisting or preventing reproduction but are profoundly affected by how children are treated.
LEWIS WOLPERT, *THE INDEPENDENT ON SUNDAY*, 9TH SEPTEMBER 1996

Wherever you look in the vast and complex field of ART you return to some key moral and ethical issues. At the heart lies the biggest question of all, 'at what point does life begin?' and, therefore, what is the status of the embryo at any stage of its use in ART? Related, but different, are concerns about the genetic origins of donor gametes and from what sources these are acceptable. IVF protocol has enabled a range of research procedures including genetic diagnosis, embryo selection and cloning. These in turn present us with pressing considerations of the distinction between alleviating human suffering by improving the health and 'quality' of human stock on the one hand, and eugenics on the other. And finally there are questions of who has 'the right to parent'? These are just some of the ethical and moral issues provoked by ART which have been vexing the HFEA and the public in recent years.

When Does Life Begin?

This is a variable depending on your religion (if any). The Warnock Report recommended a 14-day limit for embryo research, and the HF & E Act 1990 legally endorsed this. The 14-day rule has a scientific basis. Up until 14 days the embryo cells continue dividing. At 14 days (occasionally sooner) what is known as the 'Primitive Streak' appears – the first sign of organ development, which is followed by the embryo's nervous system. There are other biological reasons to support the idea of the 14-day rule reflecting a pivotal moment in embryonic development:

- Twinning by the splitting of the embryo *in utero* can occur up until 14 days.
- By 14 days after fertilisation an embryo would naturally have implanted in the womb (or the woman would commence her period) and at 14 days the embryo ceases to live independently and the placenta begins to nourish it. So scientists would argue that at 14 days a coincidence of natural activity in the reproductive process takes place, including the first evidence of a brain.

The Abortion Act of 1967 sanctions abortion on demand up to 12 weeks and has an upper limit of 24 weeks, unless the foetus 'would suffer from such physical or mental abnormalities as to be seriously handicapped'.[III] The HF & E Act of 1990 amended the Abortion Act to make it clear that selective termination of pregnancy (one or more foetuses in a multiple pregnancy being destroyed *in utero*) may be performed if the requirements of the 1967 Act are fulfilled.

The Status of the Embryo

Inevitably the status of the embryo and the foetus continue to provoke fierce debate in religious as well as secular circles. Anti-abortionists have introduced the idea of 'foetal personhood' into the collective imagination and encouraged people to think of abortion as infanticide. This is one extreme end of an argument about the rights of the embryo as opposed to those of the mother. The other extreme attributes absolutely no human status to our genetic matter up until various points during *in utero* development. Positions inevitably get polarised:

In regard to therapy, it seems necessary to accept that a large number of fertilised eggs are left to die, owing to the fact that it is common to fertilise more eggs than are needed for an embryo transfer and that fertilised eggs are selected according to criteria that one hopes to be somewhat predictive of success. An attempt was made to resolve some of the problem of waste through the process of cryopreservation. However, half of the frozen fertilised eggs are destroyed in the process of either freezing or thawing. In regard to research, it seems necessary to accept that embryos are destroyed in the process of investigation or as a result of not being found fit to be transferred to a woman. Many would argue for a definite need to do research, both for the improvement of therapy and for general knowledge of embryology. If a fertilised egg is a person none of these activities may be deemed morally acceptable. If a fertilised egg is not a person, all of these activities may be deemed morally acceptable. The early embryo is either treated as a person, or as a thing.

I think that the either-or position is false. The first attempts to claim too much, while the second claims nothing.

KNUT W. RUYTER, *CONCEIVING THE EMBRYO, ETHICS, LAW AND PRACTICE IN HUMAN EMBRYOLOGY* (ED. DONALD EVANS; MARTINUS NIJHOFF, 1996)

It is in the search for an acceptable and ethical middle ground that the HFEA concentrates its collective mind. Meanwhile, to many couples seeking ART the whole issue of spare embryos may not become a reality until you are actually told to sign consent forms. Even then, you may so fear failure to produce eggs or embryos at all that you may find it hard to have an informed and reasoned view. Perhaps now that the media has drawn our attention to cryopreservation with the mass thaw of 1996, people may feel more forewarned.

It is prudent to discuss the issue of surplus embryos as a couple, with or without a counsellor, for you will have choices to make about what to do with any 'spares': to allow them to perish, to donate them to other patients, to donate them to research or to have them frozen (cryopreservation) for your own (or someone else's) later use.

Embryos Used for Research

The HF & E Act strictly controls any research performed on human embryos. Technically speaking, an embryo less than 14 days old is called a 'pre-embryo' and any research must be performed before that time. Research on embryos must be licensed by the HFEA; a licence is only granted if the research falls within certain guidelines. Until December 2000 it was a criminal offence to:

- place a human embryo in an animal
- place an animal embryo in a human
- replace the nucleus of a cell of an embryo with a nucleus taken from another embryo or from a cell of any person
- alter the genetic structure of any cell while it forms part of an embryo.

However there has just been a major advance in embryo research regulation. With the full support of the Prime Minister, Tony Blair (who declared at the European Bioscience Conference in London in November 2000 that 'Biotechnology is the next wave of the knowledge economy and I want Britain to become its European hub') on 19th December 2000, MP's voted by a majority of 192 to endorse new regulations concerning 'stem cells' research into human embryos. Stem cells are those hundred or so cells in the embryo at 5–6 days old which have not yet begun to differentiate. They are the parent cells for all tissues, and once they do begin to differentiate specialise themselves towards the growth of the body's different parts, bones, blood, brain,organs etc. Scientists believe that if they can study and learn about the complex chemical signals which make stem cells specialise then in theory they will be able to develop different human tissue in laboratory conditions. Such tissue when implanted for example into incurably wasted muscles and organs, will revitalise growth. Using stem cells from other sources such as the umbilical cord has already proven successful as in the controversial case in 2000 of the baby conceived by IVF with embryo selection following genetic screening. Cells of his were infused into his sister's who was suffering from a rare genetic disorder bone-marrow disease, Fanconi anaemia. Her bone marrow was thus revived, saving her life (and causing media hysteria at the unfounded notion of the parents breeding a new baby merely for 'spare parts').

Stem cell research will revolutionise transplant medicine. In the future, if allied to cloning technology it could even provide us with perfect-match tissue and the growth of organs in laboratories, reducing the risk of rejection from organ transplant or the problem of finding perfect-match donors. The therapeutic potential for stem cell research has enormous potential, for curing diseases such as Parkinsons and cancers such as Leukaemia to name but two.

Needless to say, this major legislative breakthrough led to a storm of protests from the pro-life lobby and those who find the whole idea of embryonic research distasteful and unacceptable. However, the Health Minister Yvette Cooper told ministers that this extension of the existing law would be subject to strict control via the HFEA , that research would be limited to embryos up to 14 days old and human cloning will remain illegal.

Cryopreservation (Embryo Freezing)

The HF & E Act of 1990 determined that the maximum storage period for embryos should be five years, however regulations made by Parliament came into force in May 1996 which extended that storage period to 10 years. This is on condition that the genetic parents of such embryos provide their written consent. In certain specific circumstances some patients may be allowed to store embryos until a woman reaches the age of 55.

Storage periods inevitably raise ethical dilemmas. On the one hand, to produce an apparently arbitrary limit of five years resulted in the destruction of several thousand unclaimed embryos in July 1996 (embryos which the profession regretted as a loss of potential research material, and the Pro-Life lobby mourned as an act of 'mass-infanticide'). On the other hand, no time limit would presuppose no age limit for the woman eventually using them, with some mind-boggling consequences to contemplate (such as the birth of genetic twins many years apart).

Embryos are the property of their genetic parents but are under the legal guardianship of the clinic which freezes them. It is therefore essential that people who opt for freezing keep in touch with the clinic. This is particularly important in cases of separation or divorce.

What is the status of a frozen embryo? Biologically it will be probably no more than an eight-celled structure, smaller than a full-stop, frozen in liquid nitrogen. Its 'primitive streak' will not yet have appeared, and so it won't have yet formed even the beginnings of its nervous system or brain. A pre-embryo is a bundle of cells encoded with genes.

Notwithstanding, What Will You, the Parent(s) Possibly Feel about Your Embryos?

There is a fine line between regarding the embryo with total emotional detachment and regarding it as a commodity in the ART marketplace. Depending on your religious beliefs, you may find yourself thinking of spare embryos pragmatically, primarily as genetic matter for your future use. But then you may find some deep and surprising emotional attachment to them for which you may be unprepared. This isn't irrational nor does it necessarily endow the pre-embryos with 'foetal personhood'. The fact is that in the course of your treatment you will have 'met' with your own eyes some of your pre-embryos before they are transferred into the womb. On seeing them magnified hundreds of times you may feel intense joy, wonder and awe. The little blooms shown to you on the screen represent the beginnings of life which you have managed thus far to create. They are the cells of hope. Your concentration on the 'chosen' embryos might temporarily blind you to the existence of any others to be stored. That's understandable. What is also understandable is that you may later experience some kind of emotional attachment to your frozen embryos (and indeed may feel grief about any that have perished or been donated to research). They are, after all, a part of you, full of potential. That doesn't make them *literally* human.

Anxieties and Myths: Designer Babies and Reprogenetics

'Bokanovsky's Process', repeated the Director ... One egg, one embryo, one adult – normality. But a bokanovskified egg will bud, will proliferate, will divide. From eight to ninety-six buds, and every bud will grow into a perfectly formed embryo, and every embryo into a full-sized adult ... 'But alas' the Director shook his head, ' we can't bokanovskify indefinitely.'
ALDOUS HUXLEY: BRAVE NEW WORLD

ART at one end of the scale is simply practical, medical intervention to help people have babies. At the other end, by association – both scientific and imaginary – it stimulates deeply felt anxieties about eugenics. The mere idea of selecting genes conjures the idea of choosing perfections, whilst cloning falsely invokes fantasies about identical human beings created by master-race tyrants. In both cases we fear that such techniques go 'against nature'. But as regards genetic selection for example, arguably we all make genetic selections, whether consciously or not, in choosing with whom we breed 'spontaneously' (as opposed to with ART). And as regards the unnatural in cloning, Nature herself produces human clones in identical twins. To have the same genetic make-up as another doesn't make you the same person. To focus exclusively on the genetics of a human being is to ignore the enormous effect environment, experience, and education have on the individual person to make them who they are. We are nothing if not our memories.

Our profound distrust of any scientific meddling with human genes surely stems from our horror of Hitler's plans for a pure Aryan race and his disgusting use of euthanasia, medical research and genocide towards that aim. It is hard to distance ourselves from these associations. But whilst our suspicions are wise our information is too often partial and our responses reactive.

Some fear that pre-implantation genetic diagnosis has brought us one step closer to a future where children are designed in advance of their birth. They are concerned that continuing developments in mapping the human genome will mean that parents will be able to use the technology of PGD in order to choose desirable characteristics in their offspring ...

It is important to remember that regardless of the sophistication of DNA technology, genetic testing on an embryo at the pre-implantation stage only gives the patient choice. The embryos over which one can exercise that choice will still have been created by the chance meeting of a human egg and sperm – albeit in the laboratory. PGD does not involve the genetic alteration of embryos.
KAY CHUNG: DESIGNER MYTHS: *THE SCIENCE, LAW AND ETHICS OF PRE-IMPLANTATION DIAGNOSIS.* PROGRESS EDUCATIONAL TRUST. *BRIEFINGS IN BIOETHICS SERIES* VOLUME 1 SEPTEMBER 1999

We the public are experiencing future-shock in trying to adapt to the rapid advances in bio-medicine. Especially given that in the last 5 years two hugely significant breakthroughs have occurred, the successful cloning of Dolly the sheep in 1997 and the rough draft of the Human Genome Project in 2000. These two single scientific advances interact with reproductive technology and will doubtlessly transform human reproduction for future generations. But we should remember too that science moves forward in fits and starts, and the field is full of controversy. So it is impossible to prophesy accurately if, when and how this dawning of reprogenetics will enter the mainstream of daily family-making life.

The Human Genome Project

In 1990 the Human Genome Project began with the aim of completing the massive task of sequencing the 4 chemical components of DNA by the year 2003. The very (very) rough draft was completed in 2000. In its 3 *billion* letter text many remain indecipherable and whilst it *is* a breakthrough to have got this far, in reality it has been compared to finding every word Shakespeare ever wrote but not yet knowing which order the words were written in or finding all the names in the New York telephone directory and all the phone numbers but not yet being able to match them. In short, scientists are at the foothills here, far from the summit. Whilst they have a long task ahead before a complete and coherent mapping becomes a reality, we must of course ask ourselves who owns this knowledge and how will they use it? It is for example disturbing that genes involving hereditary breast cancer were patented by a US firm which has now marketed a test for them, effectively excluding any other party's research and with enormous financial benefit to themselves. It is also disturbing to learn that in the US genetic information about certain hereditary conditions might for example exclude a person from medical insurance, and even job security.

Pre-implantation Genetic Diagnosis and Gene Therapy

Against this background of global genetic research, research on human embryos to help people have babies without fatal defects has begun, with the controversial use of PGD (pre-implantation genetic diagnosis – see page 80) and the very beginnings of gene therapy. The idea that we are in sight of being able to weed out certain genes from the human stock or engineer correcting any problematic ones is what has led to the label 'designer babies' – one which might be extremely unfair on a couple who for example carry the Tay Sachs gene and, having suffered the birth and loss of a child from this terrible condition, would wish to ensure that a second pregnancy didn't produce the same suffering for all. But unfortunately this view easily offends and gets confused with having a generalised discriminatory attitude to the disabled.

It has been suggested that the use of ..(PGD)..is tantamount to saying that those affected by a particular condition should not have been born, or are less valued as individuals. Another view is that there is no conflict between choosing not to have a child with a particular condition and accepting at the same time that an affected individual should have the same rights as anyone else.
CONSULTATION DOCUMENT ON PRE-IMPLANTATION GENETIC DIAGNOSIS. HFEA AND ADVISORY COMMITTEE ON GENETIC TESTING NOVEMBER 1999

As we have seen, PGD is used specifically on embryos before implantation and in conjunction with IVF. Gene therapy – which is still at the stage of clinical trials – is a tricky procedure whereby new DNA is introduced into specific defective cells, with the aim that it will produce tissue regeneration.

Sex Selection

Doctors are empowered to eliminate embryos from the chance of life. Working in the embryology lab at King's College Hospital to create her contribution to 'The Body Visual' exhibition in 1996, the artist Helen Chadwick noted that

Like precious stones, pre-embryos are scrutinised and valued according to Platonic ideas of order and regularity. The jeweller first selects a gem for its flawlessness and then gives it additional, human value by cutting it into facets; while the embryologist examines the fertilised eggs at between two and four days, and chooses only the most clearly divided, unfragmented specimens for transfer to the womb.
LOUISA BUCK, 'UNNATURAL SELECTION' (CATALOGUE FOR 'THE BODY VISUAL' EXHIBITION AT THE BARBICAN CENTRE, CURATED BY ARTS CATALYST, 1996)

With genetic selection not only the embryo's external appearance but even its internal make-up can be 'seen' and judged.

There are two methods of sex selection, known as Primary or Secondary. Primary sex selection is achieved either by sorting sperm into those bearing female X chromosomes or male Y chromosomes or by timing insemination (it is thought that gender is influenced by timing of ovulation to fertilisation, and this can be medically controlled through hormone testing). Secondary sex selection involves either pre-implantation diagnosis or embryo screening *in utero* (*see below*).

There are 200 or so known 'sex-linked' diseases which usually only affect males. In cases of such hereditary disease where the gene defect is carried only by one gender, pre-implantation diagnosis is being used to screen out the gender at risk. There are of course huge implications. Used for medical purposes alone, sex selection carries ethical baggage. What about its potential use for social reasons? Gender isn't value-free. Cultures exist where boy children are favoured over girls, and a couple might be able to prove severe mental distress caused by failing to produce the favoured gender as a case for fertility treatment with sex selection. Sex selection could easily lead to social engineering. Theoretically at least, it would make it ultimately possible for an entire society to control its gender ratio.

Genetic screening is clearly an issue that won't go away. As researchers discover more genes, it follows that fertility experts will be able to offer patients more choice. The HFEA Annual Report, 1996 states that it intends to continue considering the technique and its ethical implications. It took advice from scientists, philosophers and groups representing those affected with genetic disorders.

Survival of the Fittest?

When the medical establishment talk about eradicating disability they mean preventing babies with impairments from being born at all. When the disabled community talks about eradicating disability, they mean the eradication of society's disabling effects.

The reality is, most impairment happens after you are born, not in the womb, so the obsession with finding-the-gene is a kind of red-herring, detracting from impairments occurring after birth and the need to tackle the disabling effects of society. My own congenital impairment was only discovered after eighteen months. Where do you draw the line? Do you start shooting babies at two?

ELSPETH MORRISON, PRODUCER AT THE BBC'S DISABILITY PROGRAMMES UNIT

Francis Crick, the scientist who discovered DNA, reputedly said in 1963 that no one should give birth to a disabled baby. Nevertheless, with the emergence of a worldwide political disability movement attitudes are slowly shifting towards more understanding of the disabled person's viewpoint. The HFEA is at pains to state in its Public Consultation document on Sex Selection that:

The HFEA considers that pre-implantation diagnosis is ethically acceptable where there is risk of a life threatening disease ... However, in reaching this conclusion the HFEA takes the view that all human beings have intrinsically equal value and on this basis deserve equal respect. People with a disease or disability have a different experience of life, not a lesser one, than those without disease or disability.

HFEA, SEX SELECTION – PUBLIC CONSULTATION DOCUMENT, JANUARY 1993
(CLAUSES 28–29)

The very notion of selecting embryos for their genetic wholesomeness understandably alarms certain people, particularly members of the disabled community. Dr Tom Shakespeare, a sociologist with the genetic condition achondroplasia (commonly known as 'dwarfism'), made a compelling film for Channel 4 called *Ivy's Genes*, about the implications of genetic screening:

Reading the newspapers you'd think we were moving towards a genetic utopia where everyday impairments and diseases are screened out and everybody's health gets better. Disabled people have every reason to think of this as a nightmare scenario.

Explaining to his seven-year-old daughter Ivy, also born with achondroplasia, just what genetic research could mean in the future, she looked puzzled and retorted,

It's as bad as saying 'you're not nice, you're not coming into this world.'[iv]

There are certainly conditions where the baby born will suffer terrible pain and have an extremely limited life-expectancy. Parents of such a child would have to watch him or her suffer and die, and clearly preventing such a child being born would be an act of humanity. The problem is, once you start screening out the genes for extreme and fatal conditions, where do you stop? What does a 'severe abnormality' actually mean? There are thousands of people born with impairments living happy and productive lives who might have been screened out at birth had the technology been available.[1] The most rational person can't help but detect the eugenicist overtones of selecting perfection over impairment. In a democratic society we may feel confident that we will keep a keen eye on the matter and never fall into the nightmare 'Master Race' scenario Tom Shakespeare and others are justly worried about. But we shouldn't be too smug. We should remain vigilant, since thresholds can easily slide. In China today, anyone with a genetic impairment has to have a certificate before they're allowed to have children. In the US a woman carrying a foetus with the cystic fibrosis gene was told by her health insurance company that the only treatment it would pay for would be a termination (the company eventually backed down under threat of litigation). Genetic information could easily lead to discrimination. Health insurance, job prospects, mortgages and the like could all be affected by people having access to health records which reveal someone to be a carrier.

The screenings offered so far have only tiptoed round the edge of the worst ethical dilemmas. The big test will come with a gene check for Alzheimer's disease ... Until last year it was thought the disease attacked at random. Now American scientists have identified the genetic factors and a risk-predictor test will be on the market within five years.
SUNDAY TIMES, 20TH OCTOBER 1994

Selective Termination ('Foetal Termination', 'Selective Abortion')

Termination can be performed on foetuses in the womb, which is why it is also known as 'selective termination' or 'foetal termination' or 'selective abortion'. It is normally performed in cases of multiple pregnancy where the pregnancy is causing risk to the mother or foetus' health, or where the foetuses themselves may be deemed impaired. In such cases, selective termination is another method of weeding out unwanted, 'defective' foetus(es). The technique has also been used, controversially, for social reasons. In July 1996 the media were scandalised by a single mother of twins who elected to have one healthy foetus aborted *in utero* because she couldn't afford to bring up two children. The Pro-Life lobby drummed up a hue and cry, and £50,000 was offered to the woman from private donations to keep the baby. By this time the operation had already been performed. In fact, Nature herself aborts many twin foetuses *in utero*. The outrage in this case was because the foetus in question was 'perfectly healthy'. Had it been impaired the woman would have certainly received sympathy, not blame. Her case highlighted the profound connection between issues of embryo selection and abortion, since both touch on the central problem of the status of the embryo, the cut-off point for termination and criteria for termination.

Cloning

In natural reproductive circumstances, offspring are a combination of genetic material from both parents. With cloning, the genetic make-up of one parent only is reproduced. Lee M Silver has compared this to creating new plants from cuttings, or splitting bulbs. So, whilst cloning *is* a procedure whereby an exact genetic copy is made across two generations, it is a confusing subject which can easily mislead us into ghoulish scenarios. Contrary to popular belief, cloning isn't 'technically speaking' genetic engineering, in that it doesn't involve the manipulation of individual genes within an individual embryo. Rather, cloning uses the technique of nuclear transfer involving the use of two cells, a recipient cell and a donor cell. The donor cell is the one which will be copied. In the case of The Roslin Institute's cloning of sheep, individual cells were taken from the mammary gland of a six-year old ewe and grown in culture in a laboratory. An egg cell from another sheep was taken and the chromosomes removed from it. This was the recipient cell. The donor cells were then injected into the cytoplasm of the nuclear-free unfertilised egg which then successfully fertilised. The sheep eventually born was the exact genetic replica of the ewe which provided the donor cells. In short, identical twinning – which can occur by an embryo splitting in two in the womb – was engineered in two generations of female sheep using *in vitro* technology.

Many IVF clincs already perform sperm injection into unfertilised eggs (ICSI), which uses the same equipment and differs only in detail from the cloning protocols described to date.

LEE M SILVER: REMAKING EDEN (IBID)

The cloning of animals has the aim of using such animals as research material for treating both animal and human genetic defects via cell-based therapies for illnesses such as Parkinson's disease, muscular dystrophy and diabetes as well as donor material and organs for human transplant. Scientists like Ian Wilmut himself (one of the scientists who cloned Dolly) is extremely wary of certain potential misuses of cloning, and intends his research to have only benign and therapeutic aims:

None of the suggested uses of cloning for making copies of existing people is ethically acceptable to my way of thinking, because they are not in the interests of the resulting child. It should go without saying that I strongly oppose allowing cloned human embryos to develop so that they can be tissue donors.

It nonetheless seems clear that cloning from cultured cells will offer important medical opportunities.

IAN WILMUT: CLONING FOR MEDICINE. SCIENTIFIC AMERICAN DECEMBER 1998

To ask scientists to stop wanting to know more, to stop them seeking to push the boundaries of their research is surely to go against their very *raison d'etre* which is to ask questions of nature, hopefully for the benefit of human experience as a whole. That isn't to say we shouldn't keep debating as a society exactly how to control bio-medical research and its application within appropriate ethical boundaries. The key factor to this is legislation, and that this legislation be brought about with the democratic endorsement of an informed and educated public.

Mankind cannot avoid change, and society cannot afford to ignore knowledge, the pursuit of which is the nature of Homo Sapiens. The accumulation of knowledge in the key area of science and medicine that led to the first human conceived extracorporeally is an example of mankind's progressive collaborative skills...once we understand what is being done, what it is possible to do, and for what purpose we should do research, then we can judge what should be done.

SIMON FISHEL: HUMAN IN-VITRO-FERTILIZATION AND THE PRESENT STATE OF RESEARCH IN PRE-EMBRYONIC MATERIAL, INTERNATIONAL JOURNAL ON THE UNITY OF THE SCIENCES VOLUME 1 NUMBER 2, SUMMER 1988

Sources of Gametes

Life can be created from the meeting of any egg and any sperm, regardless of race, religion, education or physical type. Furthermore, science is now making it possible to enter the creation game even before either egg or sperm have themselves fully developed. Eggs can be grown from ovarian tissue, and immature sperm have proven themselves capable of fertilising an egg. Progress demands that we grapple with the concept of creating life biologically rather than romantically. With ART not only are the first cells of babies made in labs and petrie dishes rather than the bedroom, but 'Man' and 'Wife' may no longer be the genetic sources of their own offspring. Inevitably this reality affronts some, rewards others and leaves the majority in a state of moral uncertainty. Traditional values of love and procreation, together with our human need to have a sense of our genetic continuity, can make us squeamish about the idea of egg or sperm coming from anonymous sources.

But many couples have no choice. Either they must accept parenting a child or children with donor gametes or not bearing children at all. If they opt for the former, they will then face trying to find donor sources as close to themselves in type as possible. This is not without its problems. Chronic shortages of donor eggs and gametes from certain religious or ethnic backgrounds cause waiting lists rising to hundreds in the larger clinics. For many couples awaiting egg donation, this can delay treatment by up to three years or more. If the technique of egg freezing had been perfected, many of these agonising problems would be solved, since surplus eggs could be donated and stored in an 'egg bank' in the way sperm is stored.

Race

In the mid 1990's there was a flurry of newspaper activity around cases of black couples who were seeking white donors because they believed that a child with lighter skin would suffer less racism. This is a terrible indictment of our supposedly multi-cultural society. It perpetuates the assumption that people are different because of skin colour and external racial type alone, when in fact geneticists have found greater variations between individuals from the same race than across the racial divide. In any case, a child born of donor gametes will not be genetically related to one or other of the people who will raise that child (that is, the person whose gametes were not used in the child's conception).

Why is a black woman giving birth to a white child any more abnormal than a blue-eyed woman giving birth to a green-eyed child, or a brunette giving birth to a blonde?

Over the years hundreds of babies have been born as a result of implantation techniques. All have been genetically dissimilar to the women in whose womb the egg was implanted. No one made a fuss about the difference. But a single case of a black woman who might be implanted with a 'white' egg has caused a national storm. Surely what is abnormal is a society that decrees skin colour is of such importance?

KENAN MALIK, *THE INDEPENDENT*, 3RD JANUARY 1994

Religion

Certain people feel adamant that their donated gamete(s) come from sources who practise the same religion. Clearly eggs and sperm are just cells and have no intrinsic religion. But we must bear in mind that certain religious groups imply racial origin (as in the case of Jewish people). In such cases, to want the religion might not only be an effort to bear a child who can remain within the faith, but correspondingly represent a desire to ensure purity of race.

Whatever motivates people in this, it is understandable that parents seek gametes that are as close to them as possible. They will probably never meet the donor (except in certain cases of DI and Surrogacy), and this search for a deep spiritual kinship with the donated gamete may be a way of salving the wound of having unusable cells of their own. It might also be a way of helping the child born to come to terms with never knowing who the donor was and having a natural quest to discover his or her origins.

Donated Ovarian Tissue

There are three potential sources of donated ovarian tissue, all of which can yield eggs for potential infertile recipients: live donors, cadavers, and foetal tissue. Baby girls' ovaries are a rich larder of eggs, containing as many as 5 million, 10 times more than the adult woman. When in 1994 Professor

Roger Gosden explained on BBC 2's *Horizon* that in the not-too-distant future it might be possible to transplant eggs from a dead girl foetus into a living ovary, or to store these eggs for future use, there was a public outcry. The 'yuk factor' was on everyone's lips. Virginia Bottomley, then Secretary for Health, went over the head of the HFEA and supported a hastily concocted Parliamentary Bill introduced by Dame Jill Knight calling for an immediate ban on such research. The HFEA held a public consultation, diligently seeking a democratic response. They got this from 9,000 sources and concluded from it that tissue could only be used from live donors in treating infertility. It didn't dismiss outright the use of cadaveric tissue, but did find the use of foetal tissue unacceptable. Meanwhile, the HFEA recommendations to Parliament that foetal eggs or embryos derived from foetal eggs should be banned from use became law in 1995.

The foetal tissue controversy touched raw nerves. Clearly the subject is emotive because it raises that old chestnut: the status of the embryo. To many people the idea of a child being born through the chosen termination of another (who would be the genetic parent) was an abhorrent conundrum. It would seem to be another case in which the medical profession and the public have different agendas: Doctors regard their job to be above all the treating of the living infertile patient. The public, looking on in an effort to assimilate the wonders (and dangers) of science, inevitably resort to generalisations and can get extremely sentimental about the sacrosanct value of embryonic human life. It is an area where issues raised by ART cross-fade into those which fuel the abortion debate. Questions about the status of the embryo seamlessly lead us to asking: 'When are human cells untouchable and when can they be viewed as human matter which might be manipulated by science to help produce new life?'

Donated-foetal-tissue-angst was also fuelled by notions of the financial threat. The Pro-Life lobby maintained that women would start having abortions in order to sell their baby's eggs off – a far-fetched scenario. The HFEA's questions to the public were more considered. Their key debating issues were scientific (concern that use of foetal eggs might increase the risk of abnormalities), moral (the effect on the child born knowing his or her genetic mother was never born at all) and consent (by law a mother must consent to her aborted foetus being used for medical research, whilst the father's consent is not needed. The use of ovarian tissue from aborted foetuses in the creation of new life suggested that the father's consent might also be needed).

The whole idea of using death to create life is actually part of Nature's own cycles. Plant and animal matter die, go in to the earth and nourish the soil to grow crops which humans eat before they in turn die and return to the earth. Dust to dust. But we don't like it when doctors play God and meddle too far in life and death (which is why voluntary suicide through euthanasia is illegal in the UK). Meanwhile, as mentioned in an earlier chapter, Professor Roger Gosden has announced a perhaps more palatable application of ovarian tissue research:

Last October I froze the ovaries of a 3 year old girl. They will remain on ice, at the taxpayer's expense, until she is old enough to have children ...
My motivations were simple; without this intervention she would have become sterile.
DAILY EXPRESS, 19TH MARCH 1996

The girl had a tumour of the kidney and was going to have radiation treatment which would destroy all her eggs and render her chronically infertile.

The potential benefits of using ovarian tissue (whether or not from a donor) from which to develop mature eggs ('egg maturation') are considerable, if not revolutionary, to current IVF technology. Researchers like Professors Gosden and Winston are understandably enthusiastic and predict that, if ethically approved, the technique could mean that in 10 years time IVF would involve a simple two-part operation costing a quarter of the current rate, with huge savings to the NHS. A woman could have pieces of her own ovarian tissue extracted when she was young, which could be frozen. When the time came for her to have children these could be thawed, matured in culture dishes, fertilised with semen and replaced in her body, bypassing the need for superovulation drug treatment, and overcoming the hazards of certain subfertile conditions such as egg deterioration from age. Egg banks would also be foreseeable, solving today's problem of the severe shortage of fresh donor eggs which blights the hopes of so many infertile couples.

Payment to Donors

Recruiting egg donors is a serious challenge to infertility workers. Whilst donating sperm is a relatively uncomplicated procedure (if a little clinical), and some men will do so several times a week, donating eggs involves medication and surgery and therefore considerable commitment from the woman donor. GLR Radio ran a programme on infertility in June 1996, in which Dr Simon Fishel of NURTURE in Nottingham reported the great success of a local egg-donation campaign, supported by high-profile media attention, which resulted in the happy fact that the clinic now has more than enough eggs to cope with demand. Dr Fishel, like many others, believes it is public ignorance rather than prejudice that inhibits egg donors from coming forward.

Meanwhile the medical profession and the HFEA scratch their heads about what to do nationally about the dearth of donors. They are concerned that, were egg donation fully commercialised as it is in the US, for example, the process might become yet another whereby poorer women abuse their own bodies for cash whilst middle-men agencies would rake off a handsome profit. Currently the HFEA stipulates that £15 plus reasonable expenses is the maximum amount of cash that can be exchanged. However, 'benefits-in-kind' such as sterilisation for the donor if that is what she wanted in the first place, or free/reduced IVF treatment, might be offered. In the case of 'egg sharing', costs are greatly reduced to both donor and recipient. Speaking semantically a gift should be free. Arguments for payment are that it is hard to find donors and that withdrawing even this small amount could be a disincentive. Ethical arguments against payment are that the involvement of any amount of money is in effect trading in the body as a product, reducing gametes to mere goods and the act of donating to a commercial transaction, all of which is demeaning and which may have adverse psychological and emotional effects on the child(ren) born in the future.

Meanwhile, both the elimination of any payment in the future and finding other models of payment are being debated within the HFEA. At a Conference on the Payment of Donors (June 1995,) some delegates suggested donors should be compensated for 'inconvenience'. Interestingly, the HFEA survey of donors published in 1994 suggested that women in the UK were not motivated by money but altruism:

The women who were surveyed were almost all motivated by a wish to help others rather than payment. They were more concerned than their male counterparts about the possible existence of children they would never know.

Whichever way you look at it, the fact remains that there is a huge discrepancy between ejaculating in a matter of minutes and undergoing a superovulation cycle and surgical removal of the eggs produced as a result. Pure altruism is an ideal, and in our individualistic and self-centred society, looking after others is certainly something to be encouraged. Meanwhile, so long as any payment is involved (even the paltry £15) I would argue that the different requirements of donor men and women should be reflected in the amount.[2]

Anonymity

Under the HF & E Act of 1990, anyone over the age of 18 years born as a result of donor gametes is entitled to ask the HFEA certain questions about his or her origins:

- whether they were born as a result of donor gametes
- whether they might be related to a person they wish to marry (or have children with)
- certain non-identifying information about their donor-parent, such as physical features, and what the HFEA calls 'talents and interests', which may be helpful to the child.

The quest to know one's origins certainly appears to be a deep human drive. Many adoptees when given the opportunity to access their birth families have opted to do so, and Adoption Agencies now recommend that children who have been adopted should be told about where they came from. So it is likely that some of this wisdom will be applied to children born of ART.

There are of course legal ramifications. Donors don't want to find themselves pestered or tapped for money by their offspring in the future, nor would recipients suddenly wish to find themselves in the midst of any custody battles. In fact in the UK donors have no legal relationship with a child born from their gametes. Whilst in the US a sad case was brought to light by the magazine *Marie Claire* of a lesbian couple who had a baby through DI with a known donor. The donor later fought a custody battle for his son and won, suggesting sexual discrimination against the women, who had actually been bringing up the child.

Age

The truth is that with the use of donor eggs taken from the ovaries of younger women, it is perfectly possible to get any human female pregnant, be she seventy years old or merely seven.
PROFESSOR ROBERT WINSTON, *MAKING BABIES* (BBC BOOKS, 1996)

Issues of age limits for fertility treatments are essentially moral rather than medical. The media's obvious delight at Cherie Blair's 'spontaneous' baby, Leo, born in 2000 when she was 45, merely underlines the double standards that operate on fertile versus infertile older women. Whilst Nature endows men with the capacity to continue breeding well into the third age, the menopause is the organic time for women to cease childbearing. The HFEA Code of Practice recommends an age limit of 55 for sperm donors and 35 for egg donors (with a stipulation that in both genders the lower limit should be 18), but recommends no limit for women receiving eggs and/or treatment. This means that decisions about age are left to individual clinicians and funding bodies.

From 1985–1995 women giving birth over the age of 40 doubled, whilst childlessness has doubled in a generation. It is predicted that 20 per cent of women born in the 1960s, 70s and 80s will never reproduce. There are obvious medical, social and economic reasons for this. Many women have elected to defer childbearing whilst pursuing a career, only to find that the price to be paid is high. Women's liberation and independence has let men off the paternal hook. Where formerly a man would be expected to stand by his mate and breed with her as a natural consequence of sexual partnership, today many men choose women as mates precisely because they 'have a life', only to find themselves faced later with the pounding of her biological clock in his ear. Such men might opt to leave the relationship or demand that it remain childless. There are many casualties of such 'choices': women keen to have babies yet finding they are infertile and/or mate-less.

Recent advances now mean that a post-menopausal woman can become pregnant and give birth as in the case of singer Joni Mitchell who became post-menopausally pregnant at 57 with egg donation in the USA, but the whole idea tends to send the public's blood-pressure soaring. A post-menopausal woman is an icon of degeneration, of someone past her sexual sell-by date, whilst a fertile man in his old age is admired for his potency, because we still confuse fertility with virility. Italy's Dr Antinori, who helped a 59-year-old British woman to get pregnant, is scorned by both the public and members of the medical profession. Most fertility doctors would refrain from treating a woman over 45, and certainly balk at one who is past the menopause (unless this occurred unnaturally early).

But hasn't this reluctance got to do with the disincentive of 'flogging a dead horse' more than anything? Clinics need success rates and older women carry a much higher risk of failure. Women's fertility takes a (statistical) nose dive after 39. This is why NHS funding and clinics operate what is essentially a discriminating policy. I say this because when people get hot under the collar about 'old mothers' and the concern for the child born to mothers past their middle age, we are surely talking of an incredible minority? Most women would choose to complete breeding by their mid-forties. Besides, the whole reason for leaving it till late in life may have been due to circumstances beyond a woman's control, such as long illness from cancer.

Dr Antinori found that post-menopausal mothers undergoing IVF with egg donation did just as well in terms of childbirth complications as a matched group of younger women. In the case of the 59-year-old woman, which aroused such media indignation, her partner was in fact 20 years younger than her, and she was a millionairess, both facts which suggest there were more than adequate human and financial resources to protect the child's future. It is perhaps no coincidence that when I scoured literature on the subject I found it was a woman doctor who came up with (rare) support for the post-menopausal mother:

I think the gut reaction to this age issue is almost an aesthetic one ... the idea of wrinklies with babies at their breasts is somehow tacky and unpleasant. This seems to me desperately unfair ... There [is a] very small minority of women who want postmenopausal fertility treatment. For those few who do it, it can be for a number of reasons. They may want a baby perhaps because they've been unable to reconcile themselves to the loss of another child, or they've been ill and they have missed the boat biologically. They may have been infertile for years due to illness, but when cured can turn from being a chronic invalid to a perfectly healthy normal woman, who now wants to do what the vast majority of perfectly normal healthy women want to do, and that's have a baby.
DR GILL LOCKWOOD, CLINICAL RESEARCH FELLOW IN INFERTILITY, JOHN RADCLIFFE HOSPITAL, OXFORD, QUOTED IN *BEATING THE BIOLOGICAL CLOCK* (PAMELA ARMSTRONG; HEADLINE BOOKS, 1996)

A relaxation of attitudes to the older infertile woman isn't exactly going to flood our society with white-haired mums pushing a pram in one hand and a zimmer frame in the other, then dying off before their offspring make it to secondary school. Older mothers are mature people who have lived a full life. If they seek a family at a later stage in life than most, they are highly likely to be able to offer the child(ren) more security, both emotionally and financially, than a younger woman can. The pregnancy will have been carefully considered and probably striven for, and any child born to such a woman will be lucky to come into life so deeply wanted.

He smiled at their incredulous wonder, and with a swift confiding movement, turned to Grandma and pulled the folds of her apron around him. He rested tranquilly against her knees while the old couple sat spellbound. Long they remained, silent and motionless, but with hope slowly rising in their hearts that Buddha had at last relented and sent a child to them in the evening of their days.

THE PEACH BOY, JAPANESE TALES AND LEGENDS (EDS HELEN AND WILLIAM MCALPINE; OXFORD UNIVERSITY PRESS, 1958)

Who Has the Right to Treatment? The Problem of Interpreting HFEA Ethical Guidelines

In his recent speech to Public Forum *Reproductive Technology: the real issues*, John Parsons of King's College Hospital outlined ethical problems presented by the HFEA to doctors and hospital ethics committees. He stressed that in one of the central issues of the whole field – patient selection – the statement that refers to 'the welfare of the child' is an instruction with no guidelines for its implementation. How do you glean information about the couple, and where from? The couple themselves? Their GP? The counsellor? An outside psychology professional? The police? Parsons summed up the only strategy possible 'on the ground' of an Assisted Conception Unit:

Over the last five years since the Act went through parliament we've had to develop our own response ... We have to be obeying the law and we have to be reasonable in what we do.

JOHN PARSONS, 'ETHICS IN AN ASSISTED CONCEPTION UNIT', TALK GIVEN TO PUBLIC FORUM *REPRODUCTIVE TECHNOLOGY: THE REAL ISSUES* (PROGRESS EDUCATIONAL TRUST, 19TH MARCH 1996)

There are many examples of where individual cases present doctors and their ethics committees with ethical dilemmas. So the current situation throughout the UK is that, just as with funding and provision, when it comes to key questions such as eligibility for treatment, there are actually no hard-and-fast rules. Interpretation of HFEA guidelines will vary from clinic to clinic. The treatment of lesbian couples and single women is a case in point. The HFEA guidelines recommend the presence of a father in the child's life, but leave the matter at that. A tiny proportion of clinics have chosen to interpret this loophole as cause for offering treatment to single women and lesbians, probably to do with the clinicians' and ethics committees' own views on the matter. King's College Hospital in London are rare in their liberality on this. Parsons described how a decision to treat such women might be reached in his unit:

Our ethics committee doesn't ask us to take single women along to them for decision making. Clearly, when we are treating single women, it boils down to making sure they have a realistic understanding of what it is like bringing up a child. Other than the counselling to confirm that they do have realistic expectations, we don't ask any more of them. With lesbian couples it is the same sort of situation. We ask for counselling. We like to confirm that the two women involved understand what they are getting into. We also, because of our obligation under the Act, like to know that there will be men in these children's lives. They don't have to have a father, but they should at least have a male influence in their lives.
JOHN PARSONS, AS ABOVE

Progress

For anyone reading this book who is concerned with furthering their knowledge in the ethical field of ART, as well as wishing to obtain more in-depth biomedical information than is possible to give here, I highly recommend you contacting PROGRESS Educational Trust. Their stated policy is:

to improve public understanding and to enhance public appreciation of reproductive and genetic science.

Their activities include producing educational materials, hosting conferences and lectures, and friends receive a newsletter and copies of their excellent annual PROGRESS in REPRODUCTION. To become a Friend costs £20 per annum. *See Addresses section* for how to contact them.

(III) Religion

Even in a society like ours, governed by secular law, the views of religious communities can exert enormous pressure on civil authorities. Bioethical concepts such as the status of the embryo are thrust, sometimes extremely graphically, into the public arena, forcing debate and sometimes changes in legislation. Abortion continues to be a vexed issue, and with the recent resurgence of Christian fundamentalism we have even witnessed murder (in the US) in the name of the unborn child. But this is only one perspective, and an extreme one at that. As we shall see, different religions come to terms in various and sometimes surprising ways with the moral and ethical implications of ART.

Sammy Lee attributes the range of religious views to a fundamental difference between a Western paradigm which has a linear view of life ('you only get one chance'), and the Eastern one which tends to see life as cyclical, with reincarnation offering the soul continuity and the chance that you can be reborn.[v] In the former, great anxiety is provoked by the medicalisation of procreation: doctors are seen to usurp God's role. In the latter the whole idea of being part of a continuum with this chance of rebirth appears to relax the relationship to medical intervention. Certainly the huge divergence of opinion between a Buddhist and a Catholic view on aspects of ART would bear out this argument. Meanwhile, the complicity between religion and patriarchal power becomes evident as ART pushes issues of parental ownership, the superior status of the male as opposed to the female and the desire for (male) genetic continuity into the foreground.

Deep in the heart of most religions is a patriarchal perspective in which the male's capacity to reproduce himself is paramount and the production of male heirs highly desirable. In 'normal' conjugal circumstances, a man would take a wife and through sex achieve this continuum of reproducing his own genes. With the advent of ART, however, sex is suddenly redundant. The man is no longer in control of his own reproduction and must yield to the greater powers of the clinicians. He won't be able to deny his own subfertility and blame it on the woman. He will be required to produce semen, on schedule and in a controlled environment. To men of certain religious persuasions this act of masturbation is a violation of their most deeply held beliefs. There are taboos against masturbation throughout Africa, amongst Arab countries, and in Catholic and Jewish communities. So a religious taboo, even if not at the forefront of a couple's mind, can add enormous stress to the proceedings of infertility diagnosis and treatment.

Another area of deep concern and anxiety is the use of donor gametes. To many cultures, impregnating a woman with another man's sperm is quite simply an act of adultery, whilst the use of donor eggs poses all kinds of questions around parental roles, genealogy and law. Some people can justify any aspect of ART on religious grounds, whilst others raise their fists in fury at the arrogance of a medical profession that believes it has the right to act like God in matters of reproduction.

Even libertarians with no religion dominating their thoughts may find themselves searching for spiritual, ethical and moral values to abide by in the daunting process of ART. The medical profession seems so techno-happy, it can be hard if you aren't a card-carrying member of a mainstream church to identify and articulate some of your deepest fears, anxieties and dilemmas and bring them into the consulting room. You may need to consult a religious person, or you may find a good counsellor who can help. It is vital that you are clear and happy about any spiritual, moral or ethical issues that may arise as a result of your treatment.

Whilst the HFEA tries to steer a course that is considered, pragmatic and consonant with the spirit of British law in general, there are many extremely perplexing issues at the core of ART which will probably never go away. Such knotty problems are the continuing evidence of a fundamental conflict between scientific and religious thought. Even when it gets hot people don't get out of this particular kitchen. Instead they take up polarised positions, the one side arguing emotively from what they see as an ethical standpoint, the other coolly appearing to regard our bodily fluids and genetic material as mere ingredients for the petrie dish. Most of us probably fumble between the spiritual and the scientific in our quest for a baby. Many of us will find ourselves making more concessions to technology than we could ever have imagined prior to treatment. We do so through force of necessity. Also because from the outside the fertility temple, staring coldly at the facts, it is all too easy to pontificate. Once inside you soon discover you are less squeamish, more tolerant and robust enough to withstand many of the shocks that ART might present you with. Quite simply, you start to understand. And on a very profound level, you start to confront many of your own deeply held views and feelings, which are likely to originate in the dominant religious perspective with which you grew up.

A Brief Summary of Religious Views on ART

> It is important to note that ART is challenging some religious institutions to re-examine their traditional views. For example, there is as yet no definitive Rabbinical pronouncement on issues arising from reproductive technology … whilst the Anglican Church has very recently stated how on many issues divergent opinions currently co-exist within the institution.[vi]

This list is by no means exhaustive nor comprehensive. It is meant as a rough guide to some of the key thoughts embedded in some of the larger religious groups in the UK. Exclusion of any religion is for reasons of space not prejudice. If you want to know more about the religious view on ART in your own faith, consult your church leader. Some religions (such as the Jewish and Catholic) have family planning counsellors whose job it is to help you negotiate your fertility problems in the context of your church or faith.

Christian

To a Christian of whatever persuasion, marriage does not have to be
validated by the production of children. The Bible is, after all, full of 'barren'
couples who are sometimes 'blessed by God' (as in the case of the Virgin
Mary). The important thing for a Christian couple is that they don't
undermine the family or rebel against God. Different branches of
Christianity have diverse views on the subject of ART:

The Catholic church holds the most extreme position, with the Pope
condemning ART outright in his eleventh encyclical 'Evangelium Vitae –
(The Gospel of Life)' along with embryo research and prenatal diagnosis.
The Pope reaffirms the long-held Catholic view that human life begins at
fertilisation. The Catholic creed abhors non-coital reproduction to the
extent of advocating making it a crime. Thus DI is condemned since it is
adulterous (involving masturbation) and is viewed as damaging to personal
relationships. The Vatican doesn't either accept egg donation, nor surrogacy,
because these are seen to offend the essential unity of marriage and the
dignity of procreation. Cryopreservation is also an offence, since the embryo
– which is sacrosanct – is deprived of maternal nurture. 'Natural' IVF,
without drugs but with a single embryo fertilised outside the body, is
permissible, however, since it involves no wastage of embryos.

The Eastern Orthodox Christian church supports medical and surgical
therapies for infertility but rejects IVF. DI is viewed as adulterous and egg
donation is forbidden. Like the Catholic church, it abhors surrogacy,
cryopreservation and embryo research.

Protestant and Anglican branches of Christianity accept ART if gametes
are derived from the (married) couple and no damage is done to embryos.
The Protestant Church finds DI morally illicit, whilst the Anglican Church
accepts masturbation as a method of semen collection for both DI and IVF.
Currently in the Anglican Church (via its Board for Social Responsibility),
egg donation, surrogacy, cryopreservation and embryo research are all being
debated. Because this church accepts interfering with Nature in terms of
contraception, some members favour applying its evolved thinking on birth
control to issues of gamete donation and its implications on marriage.
Central to the Anglican debate is the fact that, unlike the Catholic church,
church members cannot agree on the status of the embryo in its early
development. However, there are matters of broad principle on which the
Anglican Church finds consensus and which influence all thinking as

regards ART. These are, in a nutshell: a commitment to the unity of marriage and the integrity of the family, respect for human life and the principle of consent in all areas.

Jewish

The Jewish faith includes a wide range of thinking and different branches, each with varying degrees of orthodoxy. The following is a thumbnail sketch of current Jewish opinion in its broadest sense:

God's first commandment to Adam was 'Be fruitful and multiply' (Genesis 1:28), and there is an expectation on a married couple to produce children. According to the Hebrew law (the Halakha) the couple should be treated as a single unit. Fertility investigations should be conducted first on the woman; only when no female factor has been found should the man be investigated. In principle, IVF is acceptable provided it is with both the husband's and wife's gametes. Donor insemination is permissible but only in cases of chronic male infertility or when the male is carrying a genetic disease. The questions posed by DI in the Halakha are: Does DI constitute adultery? What is the status of the offspring? What about the problems of inheritance and the incest taboo?

To eliminate genealogical complications and to circumvent the masturbation taboo, DI is forbidden with Jewish semen. This means that the child will be born of gentile seed and consequently seen as pagan (blemished). If the child is a girl, she will be forbidden to marry a Cohen (priest).

Debate continues in the Jewish communities on many of the issues raised by ART. For instance, some believe the child born of donor semen is the child of the donor father, whilst others agree with HFEA rules that no legal relationship exists. At a government level, The Ministry of Health in Israel permits DI in special circumstances. As for egg donation, this is permissible although it also poses problems of parenthood. If the egg isn't Jewish, can the child be born a Jew? By Jewish law the child is related to the mother who gives birth to that child. In full surrogacy this problem is complicated by the fact that the mother who gives birth is viewed as the child's mother.

As regards cryopreservation and embryo research, freezing of embryos is permitted so long as the father's identity is maintained and there is no severance of the relationship between himself and the embryo(s). Research on embryos is permissible if it is in the interests of the father who contributed his semen to them, but the destruction of viable embryos is forbidden.

Islam

The Koran states that to have a child is a blessing from God, and consequently the pursuit of fertility is not only desirable but a religious duty. Thus fertility treatment is entirely legitimate so long as it is conducted within the confines of marriage itself. The use of donor gametes is not acceptable and DI is strictly condemned as a form of adultery. Concern for genealogical purity is threatened by the legalised 'lie' in the HF & E Act, which states that a child born of DI is registered as the offspring of the recipient couple. The taboo against any third party becoming involved in the marriage is reflected in the forbidding of egg donation. Cryopreservation (of married couple's embryo[s]) is acceptable, as is embryo research, since this is viewed as being in the pursuit of increased knowledge.

Hindu

Hindu religious views influence people via thought more than through any institutionalised values. Hindu thought which relates to infertility includes: the idea that marriage is sacrosanct, that male infertility is no grounds for divorce, and that there is an overriding duty to create male offspring. The latter means that in cases of male infertility it is perfectly acceptable for the wife to have sexual intercourse with a male relative of her husband in the pursuit of creating a (male) child. She is permitted to do this either eight years after infertility has been established or 11 years after exclusively birthing girls. As a consequence of this pressure to produce male heirs both IVF and DI are permissible (so long as the semen is donated by a relative of the husband). Egg donation is acceptable, as is surrogacy, although legal and family complications may result (not to mention the problem if a female baby is born instead of a male). Cryopreservation and embryo freezing are allowed since there is no linear concept of the soul's beginning.

Buddhist

The Buddhist faith imposes all its rigours and tests on its priests, whilst laypeople enjoy a comparatively relaxed and individualistic approach to life and death. Buddhists talk of acceptance and of the natural cycles of death and regeneration, which might lead one to suppose that they would recommend non-interference in reproductive problems. But this is not so. Essential concepts of individual freedom permit use of fertility treatment so long as it causes no harm to others, whilst the issue of wasting surplus embryos is a source of spiritual dilemma. Treatment is permissible for both married and unmarried couples. IVF is acceptable, as is DI. Whilst there is no taboo against masturbation, restraint would be advised as far as possible. Egg donation is acceptable, as is surrogacy – although, as with other faiths, it can lead to family and legal complications. Cryopreservation is also acceptable, and embryo research, since life is viewed as a process of constant reincarnation.

> The universal declaration of human rights has recognised the right of each individual to make decisions regarding his or her reproduction. Religious authorities, despite the powerful influence they exercise on public minds, should not prohibit a therapeutic approach to infertility, which would limit the area within which individuals are free to decide.
>
> JOSEPH G. SCHENKER, 'RELIGIOUS VIEWS REGARDING TREATMENT OF INFERTILITY BY ASSISTED REPRODUCTIVE TECHNIQUES', *JOURNAL OF ASSISTED REPRODUCTION AND GENETICS*, VOL 9 (1), 1992: PAGES 3–8

ⓘ The Family in an Age of ART

The 20th century has seen the family undergo massive changes. The post-war generation grew up to rebel against the conventional family unit promoted in the 1950s, where smiling-mother-in-apron-enjoys-the-perks-of-new-domestic-gadgetry whilst be-suited-father-goes-out-to-work-and-returns-home-to-a-perfect-meal-2.5-curly-haired-children-and-dog. This cosy unit was seen as both source and agent of conservative values. To change society, we argued, we needed to do nothing less than revolutionise our sexual relationships, our notions of marriage, and ideas of what might constitute a family in which to bring up children (if that was to be an option at all). Then came Thatcherism in 1979 (a year after the birth of the world's first 'test-tube' baby) with her evangelical vigour to promote Family Life, and, by implication, women's primary role as a domestic one.

Stressing the importance of the 'strength of the family' in these difficult times is powerful because 'the family' means so much to us. It symbolises our deepest dreams and fears. These are dreams of love, intimacy, stability, safety, security, privacy; fears of abandonment, chaos and failure.
LYNNE SEGAL, *WHAT IS TO BE DONE ABOUT THE FAMILY?* (PENGUIN BOOKS, 1983)

In reality, of course, economic imperatives forced the 'choice' of the workplace on many women (whilst for others unemployment gave them no choice but a breadline State income). Alongside changing patterns of female employment, many social changes have eroded the traditional family icon, including: higher divorce rates, lower birth rates, legal abortion, and the myriad ways people have found to organise their sexual and emotional lives, either as parents or not. These include co-habitation, gay and lesbian relationships, single-parenting and communal living. To the Right, such changes provoke deep anxiety and fear that an erosion of Family Values is the root of all social evil. To the rest of the population, such social changes are an inevitable part of progress and, somewhere in this tapestry of choices,[3] ART plays its part in challenging our traditional notions of what constitutes a (nuclear) Family. If a family isn't two parents tightly bound to their genetic offspring, what is it?

Parenting

There is an important distinction between wanting to 'have a baby' and wanting to be a parent. Many people want to parent. Not all of them want to undergo pregnancy. This is an anatomical given for men, but the truth is that women exist who feel the same way, experiencing an emotional and social but not biological drive to have a family. They may decide to adopt or, if in a gay relationship, may have a child with their partner through DI. In Channel 4's *Out on Tuesday* series, a programme called 'Let's Not Pretend' focused on lesbian parenting. One woman spoke of lesbians' profound consideration for the responsibility of parenting and the welfare of the child. A baby born by DI to a lesbian couple won't be the result of an unplanned 'quickie'. He or she will have been desired, sought and striven for.[4]

Lesbian Parents

A lesbian family unit profoundly disturbs the general public. Why?
There is no evidence that two women can be less fit for parenthood than a heterosexual couple. Indeed, if mothering is women's 'role' in life (as many Conservatives would advocate), then surely two are better than one!?
A happy, secure family unit is far more conducive to a child's well-being and healthy development than an unhappy, argumentative or even violent (heterosexual) one. Also, contrary to the homophobic view of gay people as sex maniacs, you can be pretty sure there won't be child abuse from lesbian parents. The HF & E Act doesn't condemn treating lesbian couples outright but, since the Warnock committee, lesbian parenting through IVF and DI has been viewed as an ominous spectre. The statement in the Act that

a woman shall not be provided with treatment services unless account has been taken of the welfare of any child who may be born as a result of treatment (including the need of that child for a father).
HF & E ACT 1990 S.13 (5)

contains a hidden agenda which discriminates against lesbians and single women. When I asked all the UK clinics whether they would treat lesbian couples, the responses were disappointing (*see A User's Guide to UK Clinics, pages 245–75*).

In August 1996 a story hit the headlines concerning a lesbian couple who sought IVF with DI and egg sharing in the following combination: In order to maximise the bonding between the baby and its parents, one women wanted to donate her eggs to the other, who would then undergo IVF with donor sperm. This rather creative solution to biological factors was refused by the hospital ethics committee on the grounds that infertility treatment is for the infertile. Meanwhile, even the Anglican Church can see that the issue of lesbian families won't go away, and includes the topic on its current agenda for internal debate.

Single Mothers

If gay parenting causes homophobic outrage, single mothers have become the *bêtes noires* of the Welfare State. They are accused of having babies only so that they can get housing and state benefits. But in a society like ours where the future is so bleak for great swathes of the population, is it any surprise that young women have babies, even if on their own? At least it presents a future (of sorts). In any case, many women still assume a pregnancy will lead to security and marriage. It is hardly their fault if the man walks away from his responsibility. Meanwhile, single women actively seeking ART will be disappointed. The HF & E Act's 'need of that child for a father' clause and the line 'centres should take note in their procedures of the importance of a stable and supportive environment for any child produced as a result of treatment'[VII] are by implication a screening-out process for single women. Again, when I asked clinics whether they would be prepared to treat single women, the answers were almost entirely negative. For single women seeking sperm donation, 'DIY DI' with a known donor is probably their best bet. For single women who are subfertile, there are sadly few options apart from adoption (from certain countries, *see pages 188–96*).

Is the ART Family Any Different from the Norm?

Amidst all this upheaval of the family composition, ART poses enormous questions about what we might now define as The Family. A family which includes any dilution or absence of the parents' genes cannot be a family by biological definition, and becomes instead a unit determined by social and legal responsibilities.

ART separates the sexual act from procreation and splits the (to some, sacrosanct) unit of heterosexually-reproductive couple into three types of parent: the social (the ones who bring up the child), the genetic (the ones who contribute their genetic material to the development of the embryo) and the physiological (the one whose womb bears the child). Because of the number of different medical circumstances which may include any of the above, the law strives to protect both recipient and donor parent from any confusion of legal responsibility. The legal bottom line is that it is the physiological mother who is the legal parent. This is why, in the case of surrogacy, the recipient parents must legally adopt the child at birth. So however the child was conceived and born, it is the adults who have sought to create a family and who will take care of the child(ren) who become their parents.

A Return to the Traditional Family?

We may well ask: is fertility treatment an endorsement of traditional Family Values? Is Assisted Conception conning us back into the cosy idea of the family unit? Is one of the reasons ART is such a growth industry the fact that deep down we want to re-affirm The Family as the most important institution we can aspire to? There are certain feminists who would argue this to be the case, and who would say that Assisted Reproduction is merely another form of patriarchal domination. Helping women to breed with such vigour on the part of the (largely) male medical profession can be interpreted as an urge to control us, and yet more evidence of the backlash against feminism and the pushing back of territory gained in the 1960s and 1970s. Cogent and persuasive as it may be, this argument isn't necessarily helpful to a bereft subfertile woman who is prepared to undergo ART in order to fulfil a basic and quite simple desire to have a family of her own. The coincidence of Tory rule and advances in IVF in the UK is, none the less, striking.

Enthusiasts of Assisted Conception technologies claim to seek to restore marital harmony and create nuclear families in circumstances hitherto deemed hopeless. Paradoxically, this moral enterprise sanctions procedures such as egg-donation between sisters, and between mother and daughter, and surrogacy arrangements, which re-write the rules of conception and birth are effectively turning family relationships on their head.

NAOMI PFEFFER, *THE STORK AND THE SYRINGE* (POLITY PRESS, 1993)

ART is full of hot potatoes. If the traditional family represents a conservative, biblical idea of 'multiplying' and of genetic continuity, the child born of donor gametes ruptures the sanctity of heterosexual biological union so dear to the Judaeo-Christian faiths. The law says that a child born to you but with only half (or none) of your genetic make-up is still your child, so long as you parent that child and take full legal responsibility for it. Bearing children through donor eggs and/or sperm endorses the idea that having children is about nurturing the next generation over and above any genetic considerations. Such ideas of parenting aren't in fact new at all. Adoption (or non-biological parenting) precedes genetic technology and is as old as the proverbial hills. This is why myths, fairy-tales, legends and the Bible abound with stories of adoption and of foundlings.

In Brecht's play *The Caucasian Chalk Circle*, the foundling child is eventually given to his adoptive mother in preference to his genetic mother because the judge decrees that the adoptive mother, Grusha, is the fitter parent.

Singer: *Take note of the meaning of the ancient song:*
That what there is shall belong to those who are good for it, thus
The children to the maternal, that they thrive;
The carriages to good drivers, that they are driven well;
And the valley to the waterers, that it shall bear fruit.

BERTHOLD BRECHT, *THE CAUCASIAN CHALK CIRCLE* (SCENE 6; TRANS. JAMES AND TANIA STERN WITH W. H. AUDEN; METHUEN, 1960)

Parents of families where there are one or more children who have been adopted will invariably vouch for the fact that, whilst the child's genetic origins may prove important to them in later life, they would never see the non-biological child(ren) as any the less 'theirs' for that.[5]

With surrogacy, the birthing process itself is displaced from the couple to a third party. The genetic make-up of the child may be half, completely or not at all the recipient parents'. So it will be the recipients' job as nurturers which will forge their parental relationship to the child. If children are supposed to endow parents with vicarious immortality, perhaps what we are learning is that this sense of immortality might be borne out more through the nurture we give the child than through his or her genetic nature.

The Child(ren) Born of ART

So what of the child in all of these permutations? Couples seeking ART are often perplexed by what psychological or emotional affect their treatment might have on the child(ren) born. There is actually very little data on the effects of reproductive practices on children. One thing for sure is that any child born by ART will be a keenly wanted child, and research suggests that parents of children conceived through IVF are exceptionally stable and loving. The child, meanwhile, like all children, will come to a point when he or she will want to know where babies come from. There isn't much point lying and telling them about storks and cabbages or mummy-and-daddy-kissing-and-daddy-putting-his-willie-in-mummy's-tummy. Far better to find a way of telling them the truth in simple and loving terms. A child learning how very much he or she was wanted should feel all the more valued and special. There is scant but emerging literature on origins. The Donor Insemination Network distribute a book for 4- to 5-year-olds called *My Story* which explains DI (*see Useful Addresses*). Tim Appleton, an infertility counsellor for 15 years, has written two illustrated story books designed to help parents tell their children about Assisted Conception. The first, *My Beginnings – A Very Special Story!* caters for different methods of treatment, such as IVF, IVF + donor sperm, IVF + donor eggs, DI, donor embryos and ICSI. Parents choose the relevant version of the story and add that page to the story book. His second book, *I'm a Little Frostie!*, complements *My Beginnings* where appropriate and tells a story about frozen embryos. The books are designed to be read to child(ren) by their parents at an early age (3–6 years). As Tim Appleton says, his books are:

not designed to persuade parents to be open with the child/children but to help them with the question 'how'?

TIM APPLETON, AUTHOR'S INTRODUCTION TO *MY BEGINNINGS* AND *I'M A LITTLE FROSTIE!*
IFC RESOURCE CENTRE, JUNE 1996

Meanwhile, it may be useful to refer to the wealth of infertility myths and fables in world culture, signs that our forebear's imaginations found their own stories to explain the mishaps and miracles of nature.

Though I came to be your son in a most unusual way, I can never cease to be grateful for the good but disciplined manner in which you have brought me to manhood. Your kindness is wider than the horizon of the sky and your love has flowed over me with the fullness of the river that brought me to you.
THE PEACH BOY, JAPANESE TALES AND LEGENDS (EDS HELEN AND WILLIAM MCALPINE;
OXFORD UNIVERSITY PRESS, 1958)

The generations of children born of ART will live to tell their own tales:

The time had seemed endless while he had been away, but now it flew faster than the wings of morning as he told of all that had befallen him.[6]
THE PEACH BOY, AS ABOVE

1. The rejection of disabled babies, which currently accounts for the majority of children needing adoption in the UK today, could be seen as a form of 'DIY-genetic selection' on the part of parents who feel unable to cope.

2. This is not intended to belittle the psycho-sexual problems that some men suffer as a result of sperm-donation.

3. To many women, of course, the whole notion of 'choice' is laughable. Arguably, the availability of contraception and changing sexual mores has 'let men off the hook' of parental responsibility. Men can now enjoy relationships with women without assuming that this will lead to marriage and babies, whilst many older women despair of finding a suitable mate with whom to breed. We may have bought our independence at a high price. Fear of redundancy, the speed of the high-tech work environment, in short Modern Life itself conspires to impel women who have careers to work so hard and so fast that sex itself may be hard enough to accomplish, even where there is a stable and willing partner. For these women children may never be an option, or one achieved in the nick of time, possibly with the help of ART.

4. This is true of a child born of ART, under any circumstances, and is probably one of the strongest arguments for the infertile's right to breed: We don't have accidents. We only do it consciously and willingly and with much foresight.

5. This isn't true of all cultures. For example, in Russia today orphanages teem with unwanted babies because there is an enormous taboo about bringing up a child that isn't of your own genetic make-up. In fact this problem is largely connected to male pride. To adopt a child means going public about your infertility and 'the average Russian Male would do almost anything but admit to his inability to sire a child.'[VIII]

6. Momotaro, the Peach Boy, has a life to live. He leaves his elderly adoptive parents, who are distraught at his departure but know they must yield to the natural cycle of life and let him go. Momotaro has all manner of adventures, setting evil to right in the world, till one day he returns home to find the old couple sitting outside their hut, still waiting for him.

APPENDIX ①

A User's Guide to UK Clinics

England
Avon
Berkshire
Buckinghamshire
Cambridgeshire
Cleveland
Derbyshire
Devon
Dorset
East Sussex
Essex
Greater Manchester
Hampshire
Hertfordshire
Humberside
Kent
Leicestershire
London
Merseyside
Norfolk
Northamptonshire
Nottinghamshire
Oxfordshire
Shropshire
Staffordshire
Surrey
Tyne & Wear
West Midlands
Yorkshire

Northern Ireland

Scotland
Grampian
Lothian
Orkney
Strathclyde
Tayside

Wales
South Glamorgan
West Glamorgan

Notes

I have deliberately avoided two kinds of information: success rate statistics and the names of Consultants in charge. The former has been explained (*see Chapter 2*). The latter is to discourage being influenced by any medical star-system promoted by the media and encourage you to reach your own conclusions of where to seek treatment and under whose care.

Columns

1 The number of treatment cycles per year is an indication of the size of the clinic and, combined with the date of licensing, can (though not as a hard-and-fast rule) reflect the experience and medical expertise it employs.

2 NHS patients may include patients who are eligible to attend the clinic as NHS patients because of ECRs or LHA contracts with the hospital.

3 Private patients may pay the clinic but may be able to get their drugs supplied by their GP on the NHS.

4 The HFEA only came into being after the passing of the HF & E Act in 1990. Some clinics (such as Bourn Hall) have been pioneers in the field, practising ART for some years prior to HFEA licensing.

5 and 6 These are sample costs per treatment cycle (unless otherwise indicated) provided in December 2000 and are subject to change. Always check for yourself what the costs include. Ask whether the clinic offers package discounts and what commitment this entails from you.

7 Waiting lists clearly vary depending on the status of the patient (NHS or Private). These are crucial to take into account if (as a woman) you are approaching 35 years of age.

8 The question asked of clinics was whether female doctors were available on request. Many clinics don't have female doctors or consultants, but will have female medical staff scanning patients. Many embryologists are women.

9 Free professional counselling. This refers to the availability of a specialist fertility counsellor whom you can consult throughout your treatment. Sometimes this is included in the cost of treatment overall, and sometimes it will be charged extra.

10 Age limits will vary enormously from clinic to clinic. They will be influenced by NHS patients' LHA policy on upper age limits as well as by the policy of the clinic itself and the views of its ethics committee.

Always check whether the age limit refers to admission on the programme or commencement of treatment itself. Does age refer to birthday or treatment within the year age?

11 Some clinics take 'single' to mean unmarried but in a common-law marriage or long-term relationship. Others regard single women as potential single parents. The clinic's policy may be dependent on the ethics committee, and most clinics where they state 'yes' would add the proviso that the ethics committee's approval must be obtained.

12 As above, 'yes' would probably depend on the ethics committee's approval.

13 Accommodation lists may be extremely useful if you live out of town and will be needing overnight stays for key points in your treatment (for example, egg collection).

14 Amenities provided by the clinic will affect your comfort and relaxation during stressful times. Most clinics will provide tea and sandwiches after, for example, egg collection, even if they don't have their own cafeteria. Tea and coffee provision refers to on-site access. Waiting room refers to a separate waiting room from, for example, the Maternity Unit. Many clinics in city centres may not have a carpark or on-site cafeteria. Check with the co-ordinator before attending about local pubs, cafés and parking facilities or public transport.

NB: The information contained in the User's Guide is to the best of my knowledge accurate at time of publication. The author wishes to apologise for any errors or omissions, since every effort has been made to contact all UK clinics currently practising under an HFEA Licence.

	Treatment cycles per annum	NHS	Private	HFEA licence date	Sample cost IVF

Avon

Tower House Clinic
22A Somerset Street, Kingsdown, Bristol BS2 8L2
Tel: 0117 924 7152
HFEA Licensed for DI/Storage of Sperm

	250 (DI)	No	Yes	1991	n/a

University of Bristol Fertility Services at St Michael's Hospital
Dept of Obstetrics and Gynaecology
Southwell Street, Bristol, Avon BS2 8AG
Tel: 0117 928 5293 Fax: 0117 928 5290
HFEA Licensed for IVF/DI/Storage of Sperm/Storage of Embryos/Egg Donation/Transport/IVF

	1390 (DI)	No	Yes	1991	See: University of Bristol IVF below

University of Bristol IVF Service
BUPA Hospital, Redland Hill
Durdham Down
Bristol, Avon BS6 7JJ
Tel: 0117 973 2562 ext 247
HFEA Licensed for IVF/DI/Storage of Sperm/Storage of Embryos/Egg Donation

	650 (IVF)	Yes	Yes	1991	£1990 ('Package')

Dept of Fertility
Southmead Hospital
Westbury on Trym, Bristol, Avon BS10 5NB
Tel: 0117 959 5102
HFEA Licensed for IVF/DI/Sperm Storage/Embryo Storage/Egg Donation

	60 (IVF) 250 (DI)	Yes	No	1991	n/a

Bath Assisted Conception Clinic
Royal United Hospital, Coombe Park, Bath BA1 3NG
Tel: 01225 825 560
email: bacc@ruh-bath.sweh.nhs.uk
HFEA Licensed for IVF (including Donor Sperm)/Sperm Storage/Embryo Storage/DI/Egg Donation

	200 (IVF)	Yes	Yes	1994	£3000 (inc. drugs)

SW Regional Cytogenetics Centre
Southmead Hospital
Bristol, Avon BS10 5NB
Tel: 0117 959 5569
HFEA Licensed for IVF/ICSI/Embryo Storage

Berkshire

Berkshire Fertility Centre
Berkshire Independent Hospital
Wensley Road, Coley Park, Reading, Berks RG1 6UZ
Tel: 01734 505 541
HFEA Licensed for DI/Sperm Storage

	30-40 (IVF) 90 (DI)	No	Yes	1994	£1650 (excl. drugs)

Chiltern Hospital Fertility Unit
BMI Chiltern Hospital, London Road
Great Missenden, Bucks HP16 0EN
Tel: 01494 890 890
HFEA Licensed for IVF/DI/Sperm Storage/Embryo Storage/ZIFT/Egg Donation

	150 (IVF) 50 (DI) 200 (IUI)	No	Yes	1991	£1800 + drugs + screening £410 for freezing

Sample cost IUI	Waiting list	Female doctors?	Free professional counselling	Age limit ♀	Will treat single women	Will treat lesbian couples	Accommodation list	Amenities
(DI) £100	4-6 weeks	Yes	No (Charged for)	None	No	No	No	Free street parking, waiting room, no tea or coffee on premises
£180	4 weeks	Yes	Yes	None	No	No	Yes	No free parking, tea and coffee, waiting room, cafeteria
£1122 ('Package')	4 weeks	Yes	Yes	None	No	No	Yes	Free parking, tea and coffee, no waiting room, cafeteria
n/a	6 weeks	Yes	Yes	40 (IVF) 45 (DI)	No	No	No (service for local residents only)	Free parking, tea and coffee, waiting room, cafeteria
£550 (inc. drugs)	No waiting list	No (female staff available for scans)	Yes	Discussed individually	Yes	Yes	Yes	Free parking, tea and coffee, waiting room, cafeteria

NB: Is laboratory service to support IVF services provided by Southmead Hospital and University of Bristol IVF Unit

Sample cost IUI	Waiting list	Female doctors?	Free professional counselling	Age limit ♀	Will treat single women	Will treat lesbian couples	Accommodation list	Amenities
£325	1 week	Yes (1) + female scanners	Yes	45	Yes	Yes	No	Free parking, tea and coffee, waiting room
£410	No waiting list	No	Yes	45	Yes	Yes	N/A	Free parking, tea and coffee, waiting room, cafeteria. Restaurant on site.

	Treatment cycles per annum	NHS	Private	HFEA licence date	Sample cost IVF
Willow Thames Valley Nuffield Hospital, Wexham Street, Wexham SL3 6NH Tel: 01753 662241 email: yvonnepayne@nuffieldhospitals.org.uk HFEA Licensed for (including Donor Sperm) ICSI/Embryo Storage	Open-ended	No	Yes	1999	£1500

Cambridgeshire

	Treatment cycles per annum	NHS	Private	HFEA licence date	Sample cost IVF
The Rosie Hospital Box 223, Robinson Way, Cambridge Cambs CB2 2SW Tel: 01223 336 880 HFEA Licensed for DI/Sperm Storage	200 (DI)				
Bourn Hall Clinic Bourn, Cambridge, Cambs CB3 7TR Tel: 01954 719 111 email: mary.walmsley@serono.com web site: www.bourn_hall_clinic.co.uk HFEA Licensed for IVF/ICSI/DI/Sperm Storage/Embryo Storage/Partial Zona Dissection/Egg Donation/Assisted Hatching	700-800 (IVF) 300-400 (DI) 400 (IUI)	Yes	Yes	1990	£2200 (+ drugs)

Cleveland

	Treatment cycles per annum	NHS	Private	HFEA licence date	Sample cost IVF
Cameron Assisted Conception Clinic Northtees & Hartlepool NHS Trust Hartlepool General Hospital Holdforth Road, Hartlepool TS24 9AH Tel: 01429 522 866 HFEA Licensed for IVF (including Donor Sperm)/DI/GIFT with Donor Sperm/Embryo Storage	200	Yes	Yes	1990	£1300
The Infertility Unit South Cleveland Hospital, Marton Road Middlesbrough, Cleveland TS3 4BW Tel: 01642 854 856 HFEA Licensed for IVF (including Donor Sperm)/DI/Sperm Storage/Embryo Storage/Egg Donation	200 (IVF) 200 (DI)	Yes	Yes	1991	£1335 (+ drugs)
Cleveland Gynaecology & Fertility Centre Spring House, Great Broughton Near Stokesley, North Yorks TS9 7HX Tel: 01642 778 239 HFEA Licensed for DI/Sperm Storage	224 (DI) 450 (IUI) inc.drugs	No	Yes	1991	£1545 (nb: at S. Cleveland Hospital)

Derbyshire

	Treatment cycles per annum	NHS	Private	HFEA licence date	Sample cost IVF
The Fertility Unit Derby City General Hospital Uttoxeter Road Derby, Derbyshire DE22 3NE Tel: 01332 625 643 HFEA Licensed for DI/Sperm Storage					

Sample cost IUI	Waiting list	Female doctors ?	Free professional counselling	Age limit ♀	Will treat single women	Will treat lesbian couples	Accommodation list	Amenities
£400	No waiting list	No	No	45	Yes	With Ethics Committee approval.	Yes, if necessary	Choice of 4 consultants (one of which is a leading male fertility specialist).

———— INFORMATION NOT SUPPLIED ON REQUEST ————

Sample cost IUI	Waiting list	Female doctors ?	Free professional counselling	Age limit ♀	Will treat single women	Will treat lesbian couples	Accommodation list	Amenities
£700 (monitored) + drugs	2-4 weeks for an appointment	Yes	Yes	48-50 (45 with own eggs)	No	No	Yes	Free parking, tea and coffee, waiting room, cafeteria. Pub located within 200 yds.
£250	2 weeks	Yes	Yes	50	Yes	Yes	Yes	Car parking, waiting room, cafeteria
£250	NHS: 6 months Private: 2 weeks	No	Yes	48	Yes	Yes	Yes	50p parking, waiting room, cafeteria
£224	1-2 months	No	No	45 48 if eggs are donated	Yes	Yes	No	Free parking, waiting room, easy access to local pubs for food

———— INFORMATION NOT SUPPLIED ON REQUEST ————

	Treatment cycles per annum	NHS	Private	HFEA licence date	Sample cost IVF	

Devon

Exeter Fertility Clinic
Royal Devon and Exeter Hospital
Gladstone Road, Exeter, Devon EX1 2ED
Tel: 01392 405 051
HFEA Licensed for DI/Sperm Storage

Southwest Hospital for Reproductive Medicine
Oceansuite, Level 6
Derriford Hosptal, Plymouth PL6 8DH
email: jackie.waugh@phnt.swest.mis.uk
Tel: 01752 763 704
HFEA Licensed for DI/Sperm Storage

| | 200 (IVF) (ICSI) | Yes However minimal provision in SW. | Yes | 1998 | £1600 | |

Dorset

Winterbourne Hospital
Herringston Road, Dorchester,
Dorset DT1 2DR
Tel: 01305 263 252
HFEA Licensed for DI/Sperm Storage

| | 45 (IVF) 120 (DI) | Yes | Yes | 1993 | £2150 | |

East Sussex

BMI The Esperance Hospital
Assisted Conception Unit, Harrington Place,
Eastbourne, East Sussex BN21 3BG
Tel: 01323 410 333
HFEA Licensed for IVF/ICSI/DI/Sperm Storage/Embryo
Storage/Egg Donation

| | 300 (IVF) + (ICSI) | Yes (with LHA contracts) | Yes | 1991 | £2150 | |

Essex

The Fertility Unit
BUPA Roding Hospital, Roding Lane South
Ilford, Essex, Redbridge IG4 5PZ
Tel: 0208 551 7107
HFEA Licensed for IVF/DI/Sperm Storage/Embryo
Storage/Egg Donation/Transport IVF/ICSI

| | 150-200 approx | No | Yes | 1990 Licence held @ Newham General Hosp. E.13 | £1950 | |

Essex Fertility Centre
Holly House Hospital, High Road
Buckhurst Hill, Essex IG9 5HX
Tel: 0208 505 3315
email: efc@essexfertility.com
HFEA Licensed for IVF (Including Donor Sperm)/
ICSI/DI/Sperm Storage/Embryo Storage/Egg Donation

| | 425 (IVF) 60 (DI) | Yes (with LHA contracts) | Yes | 1991 | £2000 | |

The Isis Fertility Centre
The Oaks Hospital, Mile End Road
Colchester CO4 5XR
Tel: 01206 752121
email: info@isisfertility.com
HFEA Licensed for DI/IUI/IVF/ICSI/Assisted
Hatching/Sperm Storage/Embryo Storage/Egg Storage

| | ?? | No? | Yes | 1999 | £2295 + £36 HFEA Fee | |

Sample cost IUI	Waiting list	Female doctors?	Free professional counselling	Age limit ♀	Will treat single women	Will treat lesbian couples	Accommodation list	Amenities
			INFORMATION NOT SUPPLIED ON REQUEST					
£100	2-5 weeks	Not guaranteed	Yes	Under discussion at present.			–	Free parking, tea and coffee, waiting room + info sheets.
£360	2 weeks	Yes	Yes (for 1st session. Then £30 per session)	45	No	No	Yes	Free parking, tea and coffee, waiting room, no cafeteria
£235 (H) £290 (D)	3-4 weeks	No	Yes	None	Yes	Yes	Yes	Free parking, tea and coffee, waiting room, refreshments
£360	2 months depending on treatment	Yes	Yes	45	Yes	No	Yes	Tea and coffee, waiting room
£500 with ultrasound monitoring £200 without	4 weeks	No	Yes (1st appointment only)	45 (own eggs) 50 (egg donation)	Yes	Yes	Yes	Free parking, tea and coffee, water, waiting room, no cafeteria
£495	None at present	Yes (one)	Yes (1st only) additional sessions £30	48-50 (but on an individual basis)	Yes	Yes	Yes - via tourist information	Clinic opened October 1999

	Treatment cycles per annum	NHS	Private	HFEA licence date	Sample cost IVF	
North East London Fertility Services Doctors House, 40 Cameron Road, Seven Kings Ilford, Essex IG3 8LF Tel: 0208 597 7414 email: msnelfs@aol.com website: www.nelfs.co.uk HFEA Licensed for DI/Sperm Storage	60-70	No	Yes	March 1999	£1800	

Greater Manchester

	Treatment cycles per annum	NHS	Private	HFEA licence date	Sample cost IVF	
Manchester Fertility Services BUPA Hospital, Russell House, Russell Road Whalley Range, Greater Manchester M16 8AJ Tel: 0161 862 9567 email: mfs@bupa.u-net.com website: manchesterfertility.com HFEA Licensed for IVF (including Donor Sperm)/DI/Sperm Storage/Embryo Storage/Egg Donation/Transport IVF/ICSI/Assisted Hatching	350 (IVF) 500 (DI)	No	Yes	1991	£1850	
Care at the Alexandra Hospital Victoria Park, Manchester M14 5QH Tel: 0161 257 3799 Fax: 0161 224 4283 email: charmian.russell@care_ivf.com website: http://www.care_ivf.com HFEA Licensed for IVF/IUI	200	Yes - if funding available	Yes	June 1999	£1850	
Salford Royal IVF and Fertility Clinic Hope Hospital, Stott Lane, Salford M6 8HD Tel: 0161 787 4699 email: ismith@hope.srnt.nwest.nhs.uk HFEA Licensed for IVF (including with donor gametes)/Embryo Storage/Sperm Storage/GIFT (including with donor gametes)	120 (IVF) No figures as yet (DI)	Yes	Yes	1990	£1600 (+ drugs)	
North West Regional IVF and DI Unit St Mary's Hospital, Whitworth Park Greater Manchester M13 0JH Tel: 0161 276 6340 HFEA Licensed for IVF/DI/Sperm Storage/Embryo Storage/Egg Donation/ICSI/Sub Zonal Insemination/Partial Zona Dissection/Transport IVF	40 + 100 ICSI (IVF) 500 (DI)	Yes	No	1991	Free (NHS)	
Billinge Hospital Infertility Services Billinge Hospital, Upholland Road Billinge, Wigan, Greater Manchester WN5 7ET Tel: 01695 62 62 83 HFEA Licensed for DI/Sperm Storage/GIFT with Donor Gametes/Egg Donation	40 (IVF) 40 (DI)	Yes	Yes DI, IUI	info not supplied	£850 (+ drugs)	

Hampshire

	Treatment cycles per annum	NHS	Private	HFEA licence date	Sample cost IVF	
BUPA Chalybeate Hospital Chalybeate Close, Tremona Road Southampton, Hants SO16 6UY Tel: 02380 764318 HFEA Licensed for IVF/DI/Sperm Storage/Embryo Storage/Egg Donation/GIFT with Donor Sperm/ICSI/Transport IVF	500 (IVF) 200 (DI)	Yes	Yes	1990	£1980	

Sample cost IUI	Waiting list	Female doctors?	Free professional counselling	Age limit ♀	Will treat single women	Will treat lesbian couples	Accommodation list	Amenities
£350	None	No, female nurse	Yes	None	Yes	Yes	No	Free parking, tea and coffee, waiting room, no cafeteria
£235	3 weeks	Yes	Yes	50	Yes	Yes	Yes	Free parking, tea and coffee, waiting room, cafeteria + info booklets and results booklet
£350 partner (£450 donor)	4-6 weeks for first consultation	No	Yes	F/44 M/55 own eggs 49 donor eggs	No	No	Yes	Private en-suite room/ctv for all admissions (inc. EMB transfers)
£250 (+ drugs)	1 month	Yes female staff available for scans but not guaranteed throughout treatment	Yes	45	No	No	No	No free parking, tea and coffee machines, shared cafeteria, own waiting room
Free (NHS)	3 years	Yes (but not guaranteed)	Yes	40	No	No	Yes	No free parking, waiting room, cafeteria
£360	2-3 months	Yes - but not guaranteed	Yes	40	Yes - if in stable relationship	No	No	Waiting room
£250	3-4 weeks	Yes	Yes	None	No	No	Yes	Free parking, tea and coffee, waiting room, cafeteria

	Treatment cycles per annum	NHS	Private	HFEA licence date	Sample cost IVF
Wessex Fertility Services Princess Anne Hospital, Coxford Road Southampton, Hants SO16 5YA Tel: 023 8079 6980 HFEA Licensed for IVF/DI/Sperm Storage/Embryo Storage/ Egg Donation/GIFT with Donor Sperm					
North Hampshire Fertility Centre Basingstoke District Hospital, Aldermaston Road Basingstoke, Hants RG24 9NA Tel: 01256 313 324 HFEA Licensed for IVF/DI/Embryo Storage/Sperm Storage	800 (IVF) 80 (DI)	No	Yes	1994	£1600

Hertfordshire

	Treatment cycles per annum	NHS	Private	HFEA licence date	Sample cost IVF
Fertility Clinic Watford General Hospital, Vicarage Road Watford WD1 8HB Tel: 01923 217 936 HFEA Licensed for DI/Sperm Storage	As required	Part	Part	1990	n/a

Humberside

	Treatment cycles per annum	NHS	Private	HFEA licence date	Sample cost IVF
Hull IVF Unit The Princess Royal Hospital, Salthouse Road Hull, Humberside HU8 9HE Tel: 01482 676 541 HFEA Licensed for IVF (including Donor Sperm)/DI/Sperm Storage/Embryo Storage/Egg Donation/ZIFT/GIFT with Donor Gametes					

Kent

	Treatment cycles per annum	NHS	Private	HFEA licence date	Sample cost IVF
The Brabourne Suite BMI The Chaucer Hospital Nackington Road, Canterbury CT4 7AR Tel: 01227 455 466 HFEA Licensed for DI/IVF/GIFT	–	Yes	Yes	1995	£1650
Assisted Conception Unit, **BMI Chelsfield Park Hospital** Bucks Cross Road, Chelsfield, Kent BR6 7RG Tel: 01689 885 908 HFEA Licensed for IVF (including with donor sperm)/ Embryo Storage/Transport IVF/DIVI/ICSI		Yes	Yes	1991	£1825-£2075
Queen Mary's Hospital Fertility Unit Kent Women's Wing, Frognal Avenue Sidcup, Kent DA14 6LT Tel: 0208 308 3043 HFEA Licensed for DI	150 (IVF) + (ICSI) 25 (DI)	Yes	No	2000	£800

Sample cost IUI	Waiting list	Female doctors?	Free professional counselling	Age limit ♀	Will treat single women	Will treat lesbian couples	Accommodation list	Amenities

———— INFORMATION NOT SUPPLIED ON REQUEST ————

Sample cost IUI	Waiting list	Female doctors?	Free professional counselling	Age limit ♀	Will treat single women	Will treat lesbian couples	Accommodation list	Amenities
£200	6-8 weeks	Yes	No (but available at extra cost)	None	No	No	No	No parking, tea and coffee, waiting room, no cafeteria
n/a	3-12 weeks	Only female	Yes	None	No	No	No	£1 parking, tea and coffee accessible, a corridor waiting area, cafeteria in another building

———— INFORMATION NOT SUPPLIED ON REQUEST ————

Sample cost IUI	Waiting list	Female doctors?	Free professional counselling	Age limit ♀	Will treat single women	Will treat lesbian couples	Accommodation list	Amenities
£485	1 month	Not performing IVF	Yes	35 NHS / 42 Private	No	No	If necessary	Free parking, tea and coffee, waiting room, cafeteria
£480	2 weeks	Yes	1 session inc. in cost of RX	46	No	No	Yes	Free parking, drinks offered, waiting room
£250	1 year	Yes	Yes	NHS: 38 / 45 NHS self funded treatment	No	No	No	Pay & display parking, hospital facilities for refreshments and waiting room

Leicestershire

	Treatment cycles per annum	NHS	Private	HFEA licence date	Sample cost IVF	
ACU Ground Floor Women's Hospital, Kensington Building, Leicester Royal Infirmary Leicester LE1 5WW Tel: 0116 258 5922 HFEA Licensed for IVF (including Donor Sperm)/DI/Sperm Storage/Embryo Storage	200 (IVF) 80 (DI)	Yes	Yes	1991	£1200 (+ drugs)	
Middle England Fertility Centre BUPA Hospital Leicester, Gartree Road Oadby, Leicester LE2 2FF Tel: 0116 2653 023 email: icacude@bupa HFEA Licensed for IVF/DI/Sperm Storage/Embryo Storage/ICSI/Assisted Hatching/Blastocyst Transfer/Egg Donation	100 (IVF) (ICSI) 125 (IUI) (DI)	No	Yes	–	£170 (+ drugs)	

London

	Treatment cycles per annum	NHS	Private	HFEA licence date	Sample cost IVF	
Lister Hospital Assisted Conception Unit Chelsea Bridge Road London SW1W 8RH Tel: 0207 730 3417 HFEA Licensed for IVF/DI/Sperm Storage/Embryo Storage/Egg Donation/ZIFT/Sub Zonal Insemination/Partial Zona Dissection/ICSI	1400 (IVF) 100 (DI)	No	Yes	1991	£2150	
Harley Street Fertility Centre 122 Harley Street, London W1N 7AG Tel: 0207 935 2234 email: rgaswam@aol.com HFEA Licensed for DI/Sperm Storage	350 (IVF) (DI)	Yes	Yes	July 2000	£2250	
Dr Louis Hughes 99 Harley Street, London W1G 6AQ Tel: 0207 935 9004 HFEA Licensed for DI/Sperm Storage	700 (DI)	No (unless funded)	Yes	1990	n/a	
Reproductive Medicine Unit University College Hospital, Huntley Street London WC1E 6AU Tel: 0207 380 9759 Fax: 0207 380 9600 email: rmusecretary@uch.org HFEA Licensed for DI/Sperm Storage	200 (DI) 400 (ICI)	Yes	No	1990	n/a	
The Portland Hospital 209 Great Portland Street, London W1N 6AH Tel: 0207 390 8262/8107 HFEA Licensed for IVF/DI/Sperm Storage/Embryo Storage/Egg Donation/ICSI	150 (IVF) 35 (DI)	Yes	Yes	1991	£2060	
Cromwell IVF and Fertility Unit Cromwell Hospital, Cromwell Road, London SW5 0TU Tel: 0207 370 4233 HFEA Licensed for IVF/DI/Sperm Storage/Embryo Storage/Egg Donation/ZIFT/ICSI	400 (IVF) 151 (DI)	No (currently under review)	Yes	1990 (but has been operating since 1983)	£1500-£1750 (+ drugs) currently under review	

Sample cost IUI	Waiting list	Female doctors?	Free professional counselling	Age limit ♀	Will treat single women	Will treat lesbian couples	Accommodation list	Amenities
£275 (+ drugs)	Varies for treatment 18 months IVF	Yes	Yes	IVF: 40 DI: 42	No	Yes	Yes	Parking £1, no tea or coffee, waiting room, cafeteria
£400 (+ drugs)	No waiting list	No female nursing staff	Yes	42 (IVF) 44 (IUI/DI)	Yes	Yes	Yes	Free parking, tea, coffee, waiting room, free initial consultation with nurse specialist
£500	2 weeks	Yes	Yes	50	Yes	No	Yes	No free parking, tea and coffee, cafeteria
£350	2-3 weeks	Part-time	Yes	43	Yes - approval required from ethics committee		Yes	Hospitality services for accommodation and travel etc.
£250 (IUIH) £300 (IUID)	2 weeks	No	Yes	Natural menopause	No	No	n/a	Parking meters on street, waiting room, no tea or coffee or cafeteria
n/a	Approx. 3 months for new referrals	Yes	Yes	40	No	No	N/a	No parking, waiting room, cafeteria. Full NHS infertility investigation and treatment. Donor insemination. Ovulation induction.
£400	NHS: 6 months-1 year Private: 2 weeks	Yes	Yes	None	No	No	Yes	No free parking, tea and coffee, waiting room, cafeteria
£300 (+ drugs)	None	Yes	Yes	Natural menopause 49 with donor eggs	Yes (with ethics committee approval)	Yes (with ethics committee approval)	Yes	No free parking but easy access, tea, clinic, waiting room, cafeteria

	Treatment cycles per annum	NHS	Private	HFEA licence date	Sample cost IVF	
Wolfson Family Clinic Hammersmith Hospital Du Cane Road, London W12 0HS Tel: 0208 740 3184 HFEA Licensed for IVF/DI/Sperm Storage/Embryo Storage/Pre-Implantation Diagnosis/ICSI/Egg Donation	1800	Yes	Yes	1990	£1600 (+ drugs)	
ACU Chelsea & Westminster Hospital 369 Fulham Road, London SW10 9NH Tel: 0208 746 8000 email: acu@chelwest.nus.uk HFEA Licensed for IVF/DI/Sperm Storage/Embryo Storage/Embryo & Egg Donation/Surrogacy/Sperm Washing for IVF Couples	200(IVF) 150 (ICSI) 100 (FET) 200 (IUI)	Yes	Yes	1995	£1400 to £2000	
St Mary's NHS Trust The Infertility Office, Ground Floor, Cambridge Wing, St Mary's Hospital, Praed Street, London W2 1NY Tel: 0207 724 2306 HFEA Licensed for DI/Sperm Storage	75 (DI)	Yes	No	1995	n/a	
Cromwell – St George's Fertility Centre Dept of Obstetrics and Gynaecology St George's Hospital Medical School Cranmer Terrace, London SW17 0RE Tel: 0208 784 2599 HFEA Licensed for IVF/DI/Sperm Storage/Embryo Storage/GIFT (with Donor Gametes)/Egg Donation	250 (IVF) 80 (DI)	Yes (if LHA funded)	Yes	1991	£1050	
Assisted Conception Unit – Kings College Hospital Denmark Hill, London SE5 8RX Tel: 0207 346 3158 website: www.kingshealth.com HFEA Licensed for IVF/ICSI/DI/Sperm Storage/Embryo Storage/ZIFT/Egg Donation/Transport IVF	750	Yes	Yes	1991	£1200	
London Female and Male Infertility Centre Highgate Private Hospital 17–19 View Road, London N6 4DJ Tel: 0208 347 5081 HFEA Licensed for IVF/DI/Sperm Storage/Embryo Storage/Egg Donation	Less than 100	No	Yes	1993	£1740	
Homerton Hospital Fertility Services Homerton Row, London E9 6SR Tel: 0208 919 7660 HFEA Licensed for IVF/DI/Embryo Storage/Sperm Storage/GIFT (with Donor Gametes)	200 (IVF) 80 (DI)	Yes	Yes	1995	£1050	
Assisted Conception Unit University College Hospital, Private Patients Wing 25 Grafton Way, London WC1E 6DB Tel: 0207 380 9955 Fax: 0207 380 9957 email: pershal@acu-uch.demon.co.uk website: conceptionacu.com HFEA Licensed for IVF/DI/Sperm Storage/Embryo Storage/Egg Donation/Partial Zona Dissection/ICSI/GIFT with Donor Gametes	300	Yes	Yes	1990	£2000 (+ drugs)	

Sample cost IUI	Waiting list	Female doctors?	Free professional counselling	Age limit ♀	Will treat single women	Will treat lesbian couples	Accommodation list	Amenities
£300	2-6 weeks	Yes (but not guaranteed)	Yes	Natural menopause 45-46 if viable candidate with own eggs	No	Yes	Yes	Car park (paying), waiting room, cafeteria
£400	5 weeks	Yes	Yes	49	No	No	No (but in house accommodation available)	Tea and coffee, waiting room
n/a	None	Yes	Yes	None	No	No	n/a	No free parking, waiting room, cafeteria
£300	4 weeks	Yes	Yes	50	Yes	Yes	Yes	No free parking, tea and coffee, waiting room, cafeteria
£250	3 months	Yes	Yes	No	Yes	Yes	No	Cafe, parking
£510	1-2 weeks	No (but available at extra cost)	No	45	No	No	Yes	Free parking, tea and coffee, waiting room, food available on request
£200	4 weeks	Yes	Yes	44	No	No	No	Tea and coffee, waiting room
£400	No waiting list	Yes	Yes	48 (with donor eggs)	No	No	Yes	No free parking (but NCP and meters close by), tea and coffee, waiting room

	Treatment cycles per annum	NHS	Private	HFEA licence date	Sample cost IVF
West Middlesex University Hospital Sub Fertility Clinic Dept of Gynaecology, Twickenham Road Isleworth, London TW7 6AF Tel: 0208 565 5117 HFEA Licensed for DI/Sperm Storage					
Royal Hospital's Fertility Centre St Bartholomew's Hospital, Dept of Gynaecology West Smithfield, London EC1A 7BE Tel: 0207 601 7176 HFEA Licensed for IFV/DI/Sperm Storage/Embryo Storage/ Egg Donation	500 (IVF) 150 (DI)	Yes	Yes	1990	£950
The Clinic of Reproductive Medicine Private Patients' Wing, University College Hospital 25 Grafton Way, London WC1E 6DB Tel: 0207 383 7911 HFEA Licensed for DI/Sperm Storage	450 (IVF) 80 (DI)	No	Yes	1991	n/a
Assisted Conception Unit Guys and St Thomas' Hospital NHS Trust, Haydon Ward, 7th Floor, North Wing St Thomas' Hospital, London SE1 7EH Tel: 0207 633 0152 Fax: 0207 928 4639 email: frances.bailey@gstt.sthomas.nhs.uk HFEA Licensed for IVF/DI/Sperm Storage/ICSI/GIFT (with Donor Sperm)/Embryo Storage/Egg Donation	600 (PGD) 700 (IVF) 50 (DI)	Yes	Yes	1991	£1250
London Women's Clinic 113–115 Harley Street, London W1G 6AP Tel: 0207 487 5050 Fax: 0207 487 5850 email: iwc@wclinic.co.uk website: www.lwclinic.co.uk HFEA Licensed for IVF/DI/Sperm Storage/Embryo Storage/Egg Donation/GIFT (with Donor Gametes)/ICSI/Transport IVF/Assisted Hatching	600 (IVF) 500 (IUI)	Yes (with LHA funding)	Yes	1990	£995
Bridge Centre 1 St Thomas Street, London SE1 9RY Tel: 0207 403 3363 HFEA Licensed for IVF/DI/Sperm Storage/Embryo Storage/Egg Donation/Sub Zonal Insemination/Partial Zona Dissection/ICSI/Transport IVF	Approx. 1000 (IVF/ICSI) 500+ (IUI)	No	Yes	1991 operating since 1986	£2275
Assisted Conception Unit Newham General Hospital 13 Glen Road, Plaistow, London E13 8RU Tel: 0207 363 8069 HFEA Licensed for IVF/Sperm Storage	–	Yes	Yes	1991	£1000 (+ drugs)
London Gynaecology and Fertility Centre 112a Harley Street London W1N 1AF Tel: 0207 224 0707 Fax: 0207 224 3102 email: info@ifc.org.uk website: www.ifc.org.uk HFEA Licensed for IVF/DI/Sperm Storage/Embryo Storage/Egg Donation/ICSI/Embryo Donation/Sub Zonal Insemination/ZIFT/ Transport IVF/Satellite IVF/Eggs Freezing/Laser Assisted Hatching/Surrogacy	650-700 (IVF, OD, ICSI) 200 (FER) 300 (IUI)	No	Yes	1991	£2500

Sample cost IUI	Waiting list	Female doctors?	Free professional counselling	Age limit ♀	Will treat single women	Will treat lesbian couples	Accommodation list	Amenities
				INFORMATION NOT SUPPLIED ON REQUEST				
£275	3 months	Yes	Yes	44 (with gametes)	Yes	Yes	Yes	No free parking, tea and coffee, waiting room, cafeteria
£1000 (inclusive)	1 month	No	No (but available at additional cost) £35ph	None	Yes	Yes	No	Waiting room
£300	–	Yes	Yes	42	Each case is assessed individually		No (but offer recommendations)	No free parking, tea and coffee, waiting room, cafeteria
£425	1-2 weeks	Yes	Yes	41 using own eggs 50 donated eggs	Yes	Yes	Hotels	No free parking, tea and coffee, waiting room, no cafeteria
£385	1-2 weeks	Yes	Yes	–	Yes	Yes	Yes	Waiting room, free taxi (within M25) on day of egg collection
n/a	–	Yes	Yes	None (except NHS limit of 35)	No	No	No (local patients)	Free parking, tea and coffee, waiting room, cafeteria
£600	None	Yes	No	56 Female	Yes	Yes	Yes	No free parking, tea and coffee, waiting room, no cafeteria. Patient support group counselling

	Treatment cycles per annum	NHS	Private	HFEA licence date	Sample cost IVF	
Assisted Reproduction and Gynaecology Centre 13 Wimpole Street, London W1G 6LP Tel: 0207 486 1230 Fax: 0207 486 1232 email: elly@argc.freeserve.co.uk website: http://www.argc.co.uk HFEA Licensed for IVF/DI/Sperm Storage/Embryo Storage/Egg Donation/ICSI/Sub Zonal Insemination/ZIFT/GIFT (with Donor Gametes)	600 cycles	No	Yes	August 1995	£2100 (not inc. drugs and blood tests)	

Merseyside

	Treatment cycles per annum	NHS	Private	HFEA licence date	Sample cost IVF	
Reproductive Medicine Unit Liverpool Womens Hospital, Crown Street, Liverpool L8 7SS Tel: 0151 702 4123/4249/4128 Fax: 0151 702 4242 email: cmalone@lwh-tr.nwest.nhs.uk HFEA Licensed for IVF/DI/Sperm Storage/Embryo Storage/Egg Donation/Transport IVF/ICSI	1000	Yes	Yes	1991	£1755 (+ drugs)	
Assisted Conception Unit Ward 1A, Aintree Centre for Women's Health, University Hospital, Aintree, Lower Lane, Liverpool L9 7AL Tel: 0151 525 5980 HFEA Licensed for IVF/DI/GIFT (with Donor Sperm)/Sperm Storage/Embryo Storage/ICSI	300	Yes	Yes	1990	£2600 (inclusive)	
Wirral Fertility Centre BUPA Murrayfield Hospital, Pine Ridge, Holmwood Drive, Thingwall, Wirral, Merseyside CH61 1AV Tel: 0151 648 2364 (& Fax) HFEA Licensed for IVF (inc Donor Sperm)/DI/Sperm Storage/Embryo Storage/GIFT (inc Donor Sperm)/Transport IVF	85-100	No	Yes	1991	£1760 (+ drugs)	

Norfolk

	Treatment cycles per annum	NHS	Private	HFEA licence date	Sample cost IVF	
James Paget Healthcare NHS Trust Lowestoft Road, Gorleston, Norfolk RR31 1LA Tel: 01493 601 770 HFEA Licensed for IVF/DI/Sperm Storage/Embryo Storage/GIFT (inc with Donor Gametes) Ovulation Induction/Tubal Surgery/Longterm surrogate of semen/Clamid Therapy/Excicular Tracking/IUI/DI	–	Transport IVF with Bourn Hall Clinic	Yes (DI) only	April 2000	£600 NHS patient	

Northamptonshire

	Treatment cycles per annum	NHS	Private	HFEA licence date	Sample cost IVF	
Northamptonshire Fertility Service The Cliftonville Suite, Three Shires Hospital The Avenue, Cliftonville, Northampton NN1 5DR Tel: 01604 601 606 HFEA Licensed for IVF/DI/GIFT (with Donor Gametes)/Egg Donation/Sperm Storage/Embryo Storage/ICSI	750 (IVF) 300 (DI)	Yes	Yes	1991	£1400	

Sample cost IUI	Waiting list	Female doctors ?	Free professional counselling	Age limit ♀	Will treat single women	Will treat lesbian couples	Accommodation list	Amenities
£400 (not inc. drugs and blood tests)	–	No	No (but counselling available)	50	No	No	Local hotel lists available	Tea and coffee
£260	NHS: 3 yrs Private: 4 months	Yes	Yes	40 NHS	No	No	Yes	No free parking, tea and coffee, cafeteria
£135	NHS varies Private no waiting	No only scanners	Yes	NHS varies Private 42	Yes	No	No	
£475 single £950 3 treatments	none	No	Yes	45	No	No	Yes	Car park, cafeteria
£450 (+ drugs)	NHS IVF 6 months No for private patients	No (but female staff available for scans)	Yes	40	No	No	Yes	Free parking, tea and coffee, waiting room, cafeteria
£320	4 weeks	Yes	Yes	None	Yes	Yes	Yes	Free parking, tea and coffee (biscuits), waiting room, no cafeteria

Nottinghamshire

	Treatment cycles per annum	NHS	Private	HFEA licence date	Sample cost IVF
Northants Fertility Service Ltd BMI Tree Shires Hospital, The Avenue, Northampton NN1 5DR Tel: 01604 601606 email: tgnfs@aol.com HFEA Licensed for IVF/IUI/Egg Donation	50 Egg donation 400 (IVF) 200 (IUI)	No	Yes	1991	£1500
NURTURE Floor B – East Block, Queen's Medical Centre Nottingham NG7 2UH Tel: 0115 970 9490 email: george.ndukwe@nottingham.ac.uk HFEA Licensed for IVF/DI/Egg Donation/Sperm Storage/Embryo Storage/ICSI/Sub Zonal Insemination/Partial Zona Dissection/Zona Drilling/Assisted Hatching/Hamster Egg Penetration Test	600-700	Yes	Yes	1991	£1990
Fertility Clinic Queens Medical Centre, University Hospital Nottingham NG7 2UH Tel: 0115 9709 238 HFEA Licensed for DI/Sperm Storage	510 (DI)	Yes	Yes	1991	n/a
Care at the Park Hospital Sherwood Lodge Drive, Burntstump County Park, Arnold, Nottingham NG5 8RX Tel: 0115 967 1670 Fax: 0115 966 7700 email: info@care-ivf.com website: www.care-ivf.com HFEA Licensed for IVF/ICSI/DI/Sperm Storage/Embryo Storage/Egg Donation/Sub Zonal Insemination/Partial Zona Dissection/Zona Drilling/Transport IVF/Satelite/IVF/ Assisted Hatching & Pre-Implantation/Genetic Diagnosis	–	Only for NHS patients under contract with health authority	Yes	1991	£1800

Oxfordshire

John Radcliffe Hospital Women's Centre, Room 10, Level 4, Headley Way, Headington, Oxon OX3 9DU Tel: 01865 222 994 HFEA Licensed for IVF (inc Donor Sperm)/Sperm Storage/Embryo Storage/Sub Zonal Insemination/Partial Zona Dissection/ICSI/Egg Donation/Assisted Hatching	850 (IVF) 530 (DI)	Yes	Yes	1990	£1290 (+ drugs)

Shropshire

Shropshire and Mid-Wales Fertility Unit Royal Shrewsbury Hospital (North), Mytton Oak Road Shrewsbury, Shropshire SY3 8XQ Tel: 01743 261 202 HFEA Licensed for DUI/Sperm Storage	75 (IVF) 75 (ICSI) 120 (IUI) 54 (DIUI)	Yes	Yes	1994 for DIUI/ Sperm storage	(satellite service with MFS) £1100

Sample cost IUI	Waiting list	Female doctors?	Free professional counselling	Age limit ♀	Will treat single women	Will treat lesbian couples	Accommodation list	Amenities
£340	4 weeks	No	Yes	none	Yes	Yes	Yes	Single rooms, 7 day service
£375	none	Yes	Yes	49 female 60 male	No	No	Yes	Tea and coffee
£475	2 months	Yes	Yes	35 (depending on HA)	Yes	Yes	Yes	Tea and coffee, waiting room, cafeteria shared with main hospital
£400	3 weeks consultation none for treatment	No	Yes	46 own eggs 50 donor	Under review	Under review	Yes	Free parking, tea and coffee, waiting room, cafeteria. Patient info. evenings, local support network
£220 (+ drugs)	3 months	Yes	Yes	None	No	No	Yes	Paying parking, tea and coffee, waiting room, cafeteria shared with hospital
£700	NHS: DIUI 1 year, IVF closed list for NHS. Private - no waiting list.	Female staff scan, 1 female doctor in initial clinic	Yes	37¹/₂ (NHS)	No	No	No	Free tea and coffee, waiting room, cafeteria shared with main hospital

	Treatment cycles per annum	NHS	Private	HFEA licence date	Sample cost IVF	
Staffordshire						
Fertility Centre-North Staffordshire Hospital Newcastle Road, Stoke on Trent, Staffordshire ST4 6QG Tel: 01782 718 402 HFEA Licensed for IVF/DI/Sperm Storage/Embryo Storage/ Egg Donation	200 (IVF) 200 (DI)	Yes	Yes	1993	£1665	
Surrey						
The Woking Nuffield Hospital Assisted Conception Unit Assisted Conception Services – Victoria Wing Shores Road, Woking, Surrey GU21 4BY Tel: 01483 763 511 HFEA Licensed for IVF/DI/Sperm Storage/Embryo Storage	NB New unit. Figure not available	Yes	Yes	1994	£1965	
Tyne and Wear						
Reproduction of Medicine Bio-Science Centre, International Centre for Life, Times Square, Newcastle Upon Tyne NE1 4EP Tel: 0191 219 4740 Fax: 0191 219 4747 HFEA Licensed for IVF/DI/Sperm Storage/ICSI/Egg Donation/Transport IVF	700	Yes	Yes	1991	£1300 (+ drugs)	
The Washington Hospital Cromwell IVF and Fertility Centre Picktree Lane, Rickleton Washington, Tyne and Wear NE38 9J7 Tel: 0191 415 1272 HFEA Licensed for IVF/DI/Sperm Storage/Embryo Storage/Egg Donation/ZIFT						
Sunderland Fertility Services District General Hospital, Kayll Road Sunderland, Tyne and Wear SR4 7TP Tel: 0191 565 6256 HFEA Licensed for DI/Sperm Storage/GIFT (inc Donor Sperm)	150-200 (DI)	Yes	No	1991	n/a	
Centre for Assisted Reproduction Queen Elizabeth Hospital, Sheriff Hill, Gateshead NE9 6SX Tel: 0191 403 2768 Fax: 0191 403 2781 HFEA Licensed for IVF	Approx 110 cycles of IVF	Yes	Yes	1997	£1300 cycle £800-£1500 drugs	
West Midlands						
Centre for Reproductive Medicine Walsgrave Hospital NHS Trust, Clifford Bridge Road, Coventry CV2 2DX Tel: 024 765 38874 Fax: 024 763 38729 email: crm@wh-tr.wmids.ntrs.uk website: www.ivf-midland.co.uk HFEA Licensed for IVF/ICSI/DI/Sperm Storage/Embryo Storage/Egg Donation/Transport IVF/Assisted Hatching	600	Yes	Yes	1991	£1395	

Sample cost IUI	Waiting list	Female doctors ?	Free professional counselling	Age limit ♀	Will treat single women	Will treat lesbian couples	Accommodation list	Amenities
£220	NHS: 16 weeks Private: 1 week	Yes	Yes	None	Yes	Yes	Yes	No free parking, tea and coffee, waiting room, cafeteria
£420	1 month	No (but female available for scans)	Yes	None	No	No	No	Free parking, tea and coffee, waiting room, no cafeteria
£300 (but mostly NHS is free)	Variable for NHS Private: no waiting	Yes	Yes	NHS variable Private patients depends on FSH	Yes	Yes	Yes	No free parking, tea and coffee, waiting room, cafeteria shared with main hospital

—————— INFORMATION NOT SUPPLIED ON REQUEST ——————

Sample cost IUI	Waiting list	Female doctors ?	Free professional counselling	Age limit ♀	Will treat single women	Will treat lesbian couples	Accommodation list	Amenities
n/a	6-12 months	Yes	Yes	None (referred to ethics committee)	Yes	Yes	No	No facilities
£325 + £150-£200 drugs	12-16 months	No	Yes	38 NHS 45 Private	Assessed on individual basis, have not treated any as yet	Assessed on individual basis, have not treated any as yet	No	–
£350	NHS, less than 6 months	Female staff available for scans + consultation	Yes	49 egg donation 45 IVF	Yes	Yes	Yes	No free parking, tea and coffee, waiting room, cafeteria shared with main hospital

	Treatment cycles per annum	NHS	Private	HFEA licence date	Sample cost IVF	
Midland Fertility Services Third Floor – Centre House Court Parade, Aldridge, West Midlands WS9 8LT Tel: 01922 455 911 Fax: 01922 459 020 email: mfs@midlandfertility.com website: midlandfertility.com HFEA Licensed for IVF/ICSI/DI/Sperm Storage/Embryo Storage/Egg Donation/Assisted Hatching	1000 (IVF)	Yes	Yes	1990	£150 inc. freezing and storage	
BMI Priory Hospital The Fertility Centre, Priory Road, Edgbaston, Birmingham, West Midlands B5 7UG Tel: 0121 440 2323 HFEA Licensed for IVF/DI/Sperm Storage/Embryo Storage/Egg Donation/Transport IVF	200 (IVF) 120 (DI)	Yes	Yes	1991 (but operating since 1989)	£1440 (+ drugs)	
Assisted Conception Unit Birmingham Women's Hospital, Edgbaston, Birmingham B15 2TG Tel: 0121 627 2699 email: julia.arnold@bham-womens.thenhs.com HFEA Licensed for IVF/DI/Sperm Storage/Embryo Storage/Egg Donation	450 (IVF) 350 (DI)	Yes	Yes	1991	£1550	

Yorkshire

Wolverhampton Assisted Conception Unit New Cross Hospital, Wednesfield WV10 0QP Tel: 01902 642880 HFEA Licensed for IVF/IUI	200	Yes	Yes	1997	£1300	
Leeds General Infirmary Assisted Conception Unit Clarendon Wing, Belmont Grove Leeds, West Yorkshire LS2 9NS Tel: 0113 2926 136 HFEA Licensed for IVF (inc with Donor Sperm)/DI/Sperm Storage/Embryo Storage/Egg Donation/Sub Zonal Insemination/Partial Zona Dissection/Zona Drilling/ICSI	1000 (IVF) 400 (DI)	Yes	Yes	1990	£1300	
St James's University Hospital Assisted Conception Unit St James's Hospital Beckett Street, Leeds, West Yorkshire LS9 7TF Tel: 0113 2064612/2065387 HFEA Licensed for IVF/DI/Sperm Storage/Embryo Storage/Egg Donation/ICSI/IVF & ICSI with Donor Eggs/ IVF and ICSI with Donor Sperm	–	Yes	Yes	1991	£1100	

NORTHERN IRELAND

Antrim

The Regional Fertility Centre Royal Maternity Hospital, Grosvenor Road Belfast, Antrim BT12 6BB Tel: 01232 240 503 HFEA Licensed for IVF/DI/Sperm Storage/Embryo Storage/Egg Donation	–	Yes	Yes	1990 (but practising prior to this)	Info not supplied	

Sample cost IUI	Waiting list	Female doctors ?	Free professional counselling	Age limit ♀	Will treat single women	Will treat lesbian couples	Accommodation list	Amenities
£260	2-3 weeks	Yes	Yes	None	Yes	Yes	Yes	Free parking, tea and coffee, waiting room, no cafeteria
£190 (+ drugs)	2 weeks +	Yes	Yes	46	No	No	Yes	Free parking, tea and coffee, waiting room, cafeteria
£325	2 months	No	Yes	50	No	No	No	Free parking, tea and coffee, waiting room, cafeteria
£250	4 weeks	No	Yes	49	Yes	Yes	No	–
No charge	6 weeks	Yes	Yes	45	No	No	Yes	Tea and coffee, cafeteria
£400	8-10 weeks	Yes (but not guaranteed)	Yes	45	No	No	Yes	No parking, no tea or coffee, waiting room, cafeteria
Info not supplied	4-6 months	No	Yes	IVF 45 (OO 50)	Yes (if in stable relation-ship)	No	Yes	Free parking, tea and coffee, waiting room, cafeteria

SCOTLAND

	Treatment cycles per annum	NHS	Private	HFEA licence date	Sample cost IVF	
Grampian						
Assisted Reproduction Unit Aberdeen Maternity Hospital, Cornhill Road, Aberdeen AB25 2ZD Tel: 01224 840 567 email: a.r.mctavish@abdn.ac.uk HFEA Licensed for IVF/DI/Sperm Storage/Embryo Storage/Egg Donation/ICSI	ISO frozen replacements 420 fresh cycles 100 (DI) 40-50 +IUI	Yes	Self-funded	1990	£1400	
Lothian						
Edinburgh ACU Simpson Memorial Maternity Pavilion Royal Infirmary of Edinburgh, Lauriston Place Edinburgh, Lothian EH3 9EW Tel: 0131 229 2575 email: neacu.compuserve website: www.edinburgh.ivf.org HFEA Licensed for IVF (inc with Donor Sperm)/DI/Sperm Storage/Embryo Storage/Egg Donation/Hamster Egg Penetration Test/ICI/Embryo Donation/Surrogacy	250 (DI) 400 (IVF)	Yes	Yes	1991	£1400 (+ £640 for drugs)	
Western General Hospital Infertility Clinic Crewe Road, Edinburgh, Lothian EH4 2XU Tel: 0131 537 1591 HFEA Licensed for Sperm Donation						
Orkney						
Balfour Hospital Orkney Health Board, Director of Public Health, Garden House, New Scapa Road, Kirkwall, Orkney KW15 1BQ Tel: 01856 885 400 HFEA Licensed for DI/Sperm Storage	5 (DI)	Yes	No	1991	n/a	
Strathclyde						
Ross Hall BMI Hospital 221 Crookston Road Glasgow, Strathclyde G52 3NQ Tel: 0141 303 4855 email: delshaker@rosshall.com HFEA Licensed for DI/Sperm Storage/ICSI Donor Sperm/Donor Eggs/Embryo Freezing/Sperm Freezing	200	Subject to availability	Yes	1996	£1650	
Glasgow Royal Infirmary Assisted Conception Services Queen Elizabeth Building, Alexandra Parade, Glasgow, Strathclyde G31 2ER Tel: 0141 211 5511 HFEA Licensed for IVF/DI/Sperm Storage/Embryo Storage/Egg Donation/ICSI	600 (IVF) 400 (DI/IVI)	Yes	No	1990 (but operating 15 years)	n/a	

Sample cost IUI	Waiting list	Female doctors?	Free professional counselling	Age limit ♀	Will treat single women	Will treat lesbian couples	Accommodation list	Amenities
£350	Self-funded 3 months	Yes	Yes	45	Only within own geographical region on individual basis	A/A	Yes	Free parking, tea and coffee, waiting room, cafeteria
£275	2 months	Yes	Yes	None	Yes	Yes	No	No free parking, tea and coffee, waiting room

——————————— INFORMATION NOT SUPPLIED ON REQUEST ———————————

Sample cost IUI	Waiting list	Female doctors?	Free professional counselling	Age limit ♀	Will treat single women	Will treat lesbian couples	Accommodation list	Amenities
n/a	Info not supplied	No	No	None	–	–	No	Free parking, no tea and coffee, shared waiting room with hospital
£405	No	Yes	Inc of price of treatment	IVF 45 / 50 donated eggs	No	No	Yes Can be arranged if required	Free parking, tea and coffee, cafeteria
n/a	Variable	Yes (not guaranteed)	Yes	36 (to waiting list) / 40 (to start treatment)	Not at present	Not at present	Yes	Free street parking, paying car park, waiting room, cafeteria

	Treatment cycles per annum	NHS	Private	HFEA licence date	Sample cost IVF
Infertility Unit Monklands Hospital, Monkscourt Avenue, Airdrie ML6 0JS Tel: 01236 712279 HFEA Licensed for DI/Sperm Storage	6 per patient 500 in total per year	Yes	No	1990	Not offered
The Glasgow Nuffield Hospital Assisted Conception Services 25 Beaconsfield Road, Glasgow, Strathclyde G12 0PJ Tel: 0141 334 9441 HFEA Licensed for DI/Sperm Storage/Embryo Storage/Embryo Transfer (nb fertilisation at Glasgow Royal Infirmary)/GIFT with Donor Sperm	300 (IVF) 100 (DI)	No	Yes	1991	£1690

Tayside

	Treatment cycles per annum	NHS	Private	HFEA licence date	Sample cost IVF
Ninewells Conception Unit Ninewells Hospital, Dundee DD1 9SY Tel: 01382 632 111 email: annemcconnell@acuninewells.sol.co.uk HFEA Licensed for IVF/ICSI/DI/Sperm Storage/Embryo Storage/Egg Donation/Transport IVF	550	Yes	Yes	1991	£1260 £1990 (inc. drugs)

WALES

South Glamorgan

	Treatment cycles per annum	NHS	Private	HFEA licence date	Sample cost IVF
University Hospital of Wales Fertility Unit Heath Park, Cardiff, South Glamorgan CF4 4XN Tel: 01222 747 747 HFEA Licensed for IVF/DI/Sperm Storage/Embryo Storage/Egg Donation/Transport IVF	250-300 (IVF) 300-400 (DI)	Yes	Yes	1990 (but operating since 1988)	£1540

West Glamorgan

	Treatment cycles per annum	NHS	Private	HFEA licence date	Sample cost IVF
Cromwell IVF and Fertility Centre Singleton Hospital, Sketty Lane Swansea, West Glamorgan SA2 8QA Tel: 01792 655 600 HFEA Licensed for IVF/DI/Sperm Storage/Embryo Storage/Egg Donation	100-200 (IVF) 150 (DI)	Yes (with LHA funding)	Yes	1995	£1750 (+ drugs)
Neath General Hospital Sub Fertility Clinic Pant-Yr-Heol-Neath, West Glamorgan SA11 2LQ Tel: 01639 762 118 HFEA Licensed for DI/Sperm Storage *Not accepting new referrals, will finish DI treatments by June 2001	100 (DI)				

Sample cost IUI	Waiting list	Female doctors?	Free professional counselling	Age limit ♀	Will treat single women	Will treat lesbian couples	Accommodation list	Amenities
No charge	1 year	No	Yes	38	No	No	No	Free parking, waiting room, shared cafeteria with main hospital
£365	1 week	No	No (but counselling provided at cost)	None	No	No	Yes	Free parking, tea and coffee, waiting room
No charge	NHS 3 mth- 2 years Private 4-6 weeks	Yes	Yes	42 Female	Yes	Yes	Yes	Parking £1.10, tea and coffee, waiting room, cafeteria in main hospital
£300	3-6 months (less for private patients)	Yes	Yes	NHS: 38 Private: None	Yes ("with partner")	No (but under review)	Yes	60p parking, tea and coffee, waiting room, cafeteria shared with main hospital
£300 (+ drugs)	2-4 weeks	No	Yes (for initial appointment only)	50 (under review)	No	No	Yes	Free parking, tea and coffee, waiting room

INFORMATION NOT SUPPLIED ON REQUEST

APPENDIX (2)

Useful Addresses

NB: These are organised alphabetically, chapter by chapter. The author wishes to state that all information below is correct at the time of writing and takes no responsibility for any incorrect information or changes of address and telephone numbers. If you have any difficulty in reaching any organisation, your best point of contact for enquiries would be CHILD or ISSUE.
For various medical Helplines, contact CHILD: 01424 732361

Chapter 1

British Pregnancy Advisory Service
Austy Manor
Wooten Wawen, Solihull
West Midlands B95 6BX
Tel: 01564 793225
Email: comm@bpas.org.uk
Website: www.bpas.org.uk

Family Planning Association
2–12 Pentonville Road
London N1 9FP
Tel: 0207 837 5432
Helpline: 0207 837 4044
Website: www.fpa.org.uk

National Endometriosis Society
Suite 50
Westminster Palace Gardens
1–7 Artillery Row
London SW1P 1RL
Tel: 0207 222 2781
Helpline: 0207 222 2776
Email: endoinfo@compuserve.com.uk
Website: www.end.org.uk

Pregnancy Advisory Service
26 Bedford Square
London WC1B 3HH
Tel: 0207 612 0200
Email: comm@bpas.org.uk
Website: www.bpas.org.uk

Chapter 2

Association for Spina Bifida and Hydrocephalus
ASBAH House
42 Park Road, Peterborough
Cambridgeshire PE1 2UQ
Tel: 01733 555988
Fax: 01733 555985
Email: Postmaster@asbah.org.uk
Website: www.asbah.org.uk

British Medical Association Publishing Group
BMJ Publishing Group
PO Box 295
London WC1H 9TE

C.O.T.S. (Childlessness Overcome Through Surrogacy)
Loandhu Cottage
Gruids, Lairg
Sutherland IV27 4EF
Tel: 01549 402401
Fax: 01549 402777
or
4 the Fairway, New Barnet
Herts EN5 1HN
Tel: 0208 440 6417
Press Officer: 0906 557 2687
Fax & Surrogacy info line:
0870 8459048
Email: cotsuk@enterprise.net
Website: www.surrogacy.org.uk

Cystic Fibrosis Research Trust
11 London Road
Bromley
Kent BR1 1BY
Tel: 0208 464 7211
Email: enquiries@cftrust.org.uk
Website: www.cftrust.org.uk

Donor Insemination and Egg Donation
Helpline: 01278 671654

Donor Insemination Network
PO Box 265
Sheffield S3 7YX

Down's Syndrome Association
155 Mitcham Road
London SW17 9PG
Tel: 0208 682 4001
Fax: 0208 682 4012
Email:
info@downs_syndrome.org.uk
Website: downs_syndrome.org.uk

Egg Donor Advice Centre & Assisted Conception Unit
King's Healthcare ACU
King's College
Tel: 0207 346 3158 (message)
or
National Egg and Embryo Donation
Society (N.E.E.D.S)
Tel: 0161 276 6000

GIFT Helpline
Several in UK: consult Directory
Enquiries, CHILD (01424 732361)
or ISSUE

Hysterectomy Support Group
The Venture
Green Lane, Upton
Huntington PE17 5YE

Miscarriage Association
c/o Clayton Hospital
Northgate, Wakefield
West Yorkshire WF1 3JS
Tel: 01924 200799
Fax: 01924 298834
Website: www.the_ma.org.uk

Multiple Births Foundation
Institute of Obstetrics and
Gynaecology
Queen Charlotte's Hospital
Goldhawk Road
London W6 0XG
Tel: 0208 748 4666

National AIDS Trust
New City Cloisters
196 Old Street, London EC1V 9FR
Tel: 0207 814 6767

Organon Laboratories Ltd
Cambridge Science Park
Cambridge CB4 4FL

The Royal Society for Disability and Rehabilitation (RADAR)
12 City Forum, 250 City Road
London EC1V 8AF
Tel: 0207 250 3222
Email: radar@radar.org.uk
Website: www.radar.org.uk

Stillbirth and Neonatal Death Society (SANDS)
28 Portland Place
London W1B 1LY
Tel: 0207 436 7940
Fax: 0207 436 3715
Helpline: 0207 436 5881
Email: support@uk_sands.org.uk
Website: www.uk_sands.org.uk

Support Around Termination for Abnormality (SAFTA)
73–75 Charlotte Street
London W1P 1LB
Tel: 0207 631 0280
Helpline: 0207 631 0285

Twins and Multiple Births Association (TAMBA)
Harnott House
309 Chester Road
Little Sutton
Wirral L66 1QQ
Tel: 0870 121 4000
Email: tamba@information4u.com
Website: www.tamba.org.uk

Verity (Polycystic Ovary Syndrome Support Group)
Tindle Manor
52–54 Featherstone Street
London EC1Y 8RT
Send SAE, wait 28 days for reply.

For specific medical Helplines
contact CHILD: 01424 732361

Chapter 3

Active Birth Movement
55 Dartmouth Park Road
London NW5 1SL
Tel: 0207 267 3006

British Association of Counselling
1 Regent Place
Rugby
Warwickshire CV21 2PJ
Tel: 01788 550899
Fax: 01788 562189
Email: bacp@bacp.co.uk
Website: www.counselling.co.uk

British Infertility Counsellors Association
69 Division Street
Sheffield
West Yorks S1 4GE
Tel: 01342 843880
Website: www.bica.net

CHILD
Charter House
43 St Leonards Road
Bexhill on Sea
East Sussex TN40 1JA
Tel: 01424 732361
Fax: 01424 731858
E-mail: office@e-mail.2.child.org.uk
Website:
www:http://www/child.org.uk

Infertility Support Group
c/o Women's Health and
Reproductive Rights Information
Centre
52–54 Featherstone Street
London EC1Y 8RT
Tel: 0207 251 6580

Involuntary Childless Support Group
38a Chase Green Avenue
Enfield EN2 8EB
Tel: 0208 366 3075

ISSUE (The National Fertility Association)
114 Lichfield Street
Walsall WS1 1SZ
Tel: 01922 722888
Fax: 01922 640070
E-mail: webmaster@issue.co.uk

National Gamete Donation Trust
PO Box 52, Bury
Lancashire BL0 9GE
Tel: 01706 829428
Fax: 01706 829429
Email: ajmillwand.ngdt@tesco.net

RELATE (national headquarters)
Little Church Street
Rugby
Warwickshire CV21 3AP
Tel: 01788 573241
Fax: 01788 535007
Website: www.relate.org.uk

SAMARITANS
Linkline: 0345 909090

Women's Health
52 Featherstone Street
London EC1Y 8RT
Tel: 0207 263 6394

Women's Therapy Centre
10 Manor Gardens
London N7 6JS
Tel: 0207 263 6200
Email:
info@womenstherapycentre.co.uk
Website:
www.womenstherapycentre.co.uk

Chapter 4

London Lesbian and Gay Switchboard
Tel: 0207 837 7324

Survey of NHS Infertility Services 1997-8 will be available on the Internet at:
http.//www.doh.gov.uk/infertility treatment

The RCOG guidelines can be obtained from RCOG bookshop.
Tel: 0207 772 6275 or
Email: bookshop@vcog.org.uk

NIAC
PO Box 2106
London W1A 3DZ
Freefone: 0800 716345

Women and Medical Practice
48 Turnpike Lane, London
Tel: 0208 888 2782
For lesbian self-insemination groups, see Women's Health Concern, below

Also Local Health Authorities and your local MP

Chapter 5

Alcoholics Anonymous
General Services Offices
Tel: 01904 644026
Website:
alcoholics.anonymous.org.uk

Allen Carr
(quit smoking hypnotherapy)
www.allencarrseasyway.com

The British Acupuncture Council
63 Jeddo Road
London W12 9HG
Tel: 0208 735 0400
Fax: 0208 735 0404

British Hypnotherapy Association
67 Upper Berkeley Street
Marble Arch
London W1H 7QX
Tel: 0207 723 4443

The British Register of Complementary Practitioners
1 Sweden Gate
London SE16 1TG
Tel/Fax: 0207 237 5175

Eating Disorders Association
Sackville Place
44 Magdalen Street
Norwich NR3 1JU
Tel: 01603 621414

FORESIGHT
(Association for the promotion of pre-conceptual care)
28 The Paddock
Godalming
Surrey GU7 1XD
Tel: 01483 427839

Institute of Optimum Nutrition
Blades Court
Deodar Road
London SW15 2NU
Tel: 0208 877 9993
Email: ion@cablenet.co.uk
Website: www.ion.ac.uk

The Register of Qualified Aromatherapists
PO Box 6941
London N8 9HF

Weightwatchers UK Ltd (national headquarters)
Kidwells Park House
Kidwells Park Drive
Maidenhead, Berks SL6 8YT
Tel: 01628 777077
Website:
www.uk.weighwatchers.com

Woman's Health Concern
Ground Floor Hall
17 Earl's Terrace
London W8 6LP
Tel: 0208 780 3916

Women's Nutritional Advisory Service
PO Box 268
Hove
Sussex BN3 1RW

also Local Social Services

Chapter 6

Adoption UK
Lower Boddington
Daventry
Northants NN11 6YB
Tel: 01327 260295
Fax: 01327 263565

AFAA
The Association of Families who
have adopted from abroad
71 Chelsham Road
South Croydon, Surrey CR2 6HZ

British Agencies for Adoption and Fostering (BAAF)
Skyline House
200 Union Street
London SE1 0LX
Tel: 0207 593 2000
Fax: 0207 593 2001
Email: mail@baaf.org.uk
Website: www.baaf.org.uk

BAAF Adoption and Fostering NE Office
MEA House, Ellison Place
Newcastle Upon Tyne NE1 8XS
Tel: 0191 261 6600
Email: newcastle@baaf.org.uk
Website: www.baaf.org.uk

BAAF Central Region
St George's House
Coventry Road, Coleshill
Birmingham B46 3EA
Tel: 01675 463998
Email: midlands@baaf.org.uk
Website: www.baaf.org.uk

BAAF Northern Region Offices
Grove Villa
82 Cardigan Road
Headingley
Leeds LS6 3BJ
Tel: 0113 274 4797

BAAF Scottish Centre
40 Shandwick Place
Edinburgh EH2 4RT
Tel: 0131 225 9285

BAAF Southern Region
Skyline House
200 Union Street
London SE1 0LX
Tel: 0207 928 6085
and
9 Stokes Croft
Bristol BS1 3PL
Tel: 0117 942 5881

BAAF Welsh Centre
7 Cleeve House
Lambourne Crescent
Cardiff CF14 5GP
Tel: 02920 761155
Email: cymru@baaf.org.uk
Website: www.baaf.org.uk

Guatemalan Families Association
PO Box 16911
London SE3 9TG

Dept of Health Adoption Unit
Wellington House
Waterloo
London SE1 8UG
Tel: 0207 972 4082
Website:
www.doh.gov.uk/coinh.htm

Home Office Immigration
Lunar House
Wellesley Road
Croydon CR9 2BY

**Jewish Association for
Fostering, Adoption and
Infertility (JAFA)**
PO Box 20
Prestwich
Manchester M25 5BY
Tel: 0161 773 3148

**National Foster Care
Association Helpline**
Tel: 0207 620 2100 (*NB*: Mon, Tue,
Thurs, Fri only between
1–4.30 p.m.)

**National Foster Care
Association (NFCA)**
87 Blackfriars Road
London SE1 8HA
Tel: 0207 6206400
Advice Line: 0207 378 8015
(1–4.30 p.m.)

**National Foster Care
Association Scotland**
1 Melrose Street
(off Queens Crescent)
Glasgow G4 9BT
Tel: 0141 332 6655

OASIS
Coral Williams
Dan y Graig
Balaclava Road
Glais
Swansea SA7 9HJ
Tel: 01792 844329

**Overseas Adoption
Helpline**
First Floor
34 Upper Street
London N1 0PN
Tel: 0870 5168742 (Mon–Wed,
2–5 p.m.)
Fax: 0207 704 2387

**Parent to Parent
Information on Adoption
Services (PPIAS)**
Lower Boddington
Daventry
Northamptonshire NN11 6YB
Tel: 0208 348 1522

**The Performance and
Innovation Report on
Adoption 2000**
Website: www.cabinet_office.gov.uk
or
www.doh.gov.uk/coinh.htm

Post Adoption Centre
8 Torriano Mews
London NW5 2RZ
Tel: 0207 284 0555

Chapter 7

Antenatal Results & Choices (ARC)
73–75 Charlotte Street
London W1P 1LB
Tel/Fax: 0207 631 0280
Parents Helpline: 0207 631 0285

The Board for Social Responsibility
The General Synod of the
Church of England
Church House
Great Smith Street
London SW1P 3NZ
Tel: 0207 222 9011

Contact a Family
170 Tottenham Court Road
London W1P 0HA
Tel: 0207 383 3555
Fax: 0207 383 0259
Email: info@cafamily.org.uk

Genetic Interest Group
Farringdon Point
29–35 Farringdon Road
London EC1M 3JB
Tel: 0207 430 0090
Fax: 0207 430 0092
Email:
101366.760@compuserve.com

Human Fertilisation and Embryology Authority (HFEA)
Paxton House
30 Artillery Lane
London E1 7LS
Tel: 0207 377 5077

Independent Fertility Concerns
(books, CD Rom, information, counselling)
The IFC Resource Centre
44 Eversden Road
Harlton
Cambridge CB3 7ET
Tel: 01223 262 226
Fax: 01223 264 332
E-mail: fw39@dial.pipex.com

Dr A Majid Katme (Muslim Spokesman on bioethical issues)
31 North Circular Road
Palmers Green
London N13 5EG
Tel/Fax: 0208 345 6220

The Linacre Centre (Catholic Advisory Centre on Bioethics)
60 Grove End Road
London NW8 9NH
Tel: 0207 289 3625

National Council for One Parent Families
255 Kentish Town Road
London NW5 2LX
Tel: 0207 267 1361

Progress Educational Trust
140 Grays Inn Road
London WC1X 8AX
Tel: 0207 278 7870
Fax: 0207 278 7862
Email: admin@progress.org.uk
www.progress.org.uk/news

Useful Websites recommended by the Progress Educational Trust

Acebabies
Assisted Conception Babies Support for Families following successful fertility treatment
www.acebabies.co.uk

Human Genome Project Information
http://www.ornl.gov/TechResources/Human_Genome/home.html

The Geneletter
http://www.geneletter.org/index.epl

Bioethics.net
http://www.med.upenn.edu/%7Ebioethic/index.shtml

Ferti.net
http://www.ferti.net/

The American Infertility Association
http://www.americaninfertility.org/

BBC news online
http://news.bbc.co.uk/

New Scientist
http://www.newscientist.com

An ABC of ART

Abortion
Pregnancy loss. 'Spontaneous abortion' is another term for miscarriage, when the loss has occurred naturally. 'Selective abortion' is when a pregnancy, or one or more babies in a multiple pregnancy, is terminated medically.

Acrosome
Cap on the head of a sperm.

Adhesion
Scar tissue (such as after infection or surgery) which forms a band and then binds organs together.

AIH
See **Artificial Insemination**

Amenorrhoea (also Anovulation)
Female condition where there is a total absence of ovulation and menstruation.

Andrology
Branch of medicine that specialises in male diseases.

Anorexia Nervosa
So-called (misleadingly) the 'slimmers' disease', this is a psychologically-provoked condition where loss of appetite or deliberate starvation produces dangerous weight loss leading to secondary conditions including anovulation in women. Though far rarer, men can suffer anorexia.

ART
See **Assisted Reproduction Technology**

Artificial Insemination (AIH)
Artificial insemination using the husband's (or partner's) sperm and introducing it into the cervix by means of a syringe.

Assisted Reproduction (or Assisted Conception)
Collective term for infertility treatments.

Assisted Reproduction Technology (or Technologies)
Term referring to new medical technologies (including drugs, surgery, micro-manipulation, cryopreservation, etc.).

Asthenozoospermia
Male condition where less than 40 per cent of sperm are motile.

Azoospermia
Male condition where there is no sperm in the semen.

Basal Body Temperature (BBT)
The temperature of the body at rest. A BBT chart is used to monitor the body's natural rise in temperature after ovulation as a method of ovulation prediction or birth control.

Biopsy
Surgical removal of body tissue for laboratory analysis.

Birth Control
See **Contraception**

Blastocyst
A fertilised egg at the stage of its attachment to the womb lining.

Blighted Ovum
A fertilised egg (embryo) which fails to develop after implantation in the uterine wall, resulting in spontaneous abortion (miscarriage).

Buserelin
Brand name of hormone drug used to reduce the activity of the pituitary gland and consequently inhibit ovulation (used in IVF).

Caesarean Section (C-Section)
Named after Julius Caesar, who was born this way, the term refers to surgical delivery of a baby via an incision in the lower abdominal wall, with the mother under either a local or general anaesthetic.

Cancer
Malignant growth of cells.

Candida Albicans
A yeast-like fungus ('thrush') which can be found in the vagina, causing vaginal itching, dryness and discharge, and dryness in the tip of the penis. It can also be found in the mouth and in the gut.

Candidiasis
When Candida takes root and penetrates the gut wall, it can contribute to poor absorption of nutrients which is thought by some researchers to affect fertility.

Capacitation
The breaking up of the sperm's outer layer.

Cervical Mucus
Secretions in the cervical canal.

Cervix
The neck of the womb.

Chlamydia
A micro-organism found in the genito-urinary tract, which may be sexually transmitted, causing mild to severe infection.

Chromosomes
If DNA is the language of inheritance, genes are its sentences, to be found on the 46 chromosomes in any one human cell. Of these 46, 23 chromosomes derive from the egg and 23 from sperm. The sex chromosome deriving from the egg is known as an X, whilst sperm can produce either an X or a Y. An XY combination produces a boy, an XX a girl. When chromosomes are damaged, miscarriage usually occurs. Common gene abnormalities which don't spontaneously abort are Trisomy 21 (Down's Syndrome) and Trisomy 13 (cleft palate).

Chronic
A condition which is prolonged.

Cilia
Hair-like projections which grow out of certain cells.

Clitoris
Bud of highly sensitive erectile tissue above a woman's vagina.

Clomid
Brand name for the fertility hormone clomiphene citrate (oestrogen).

Coitus
Heterosexual intercourse (*also see* **Post-Coital Test**).

Colon
Part of the large intestine which leads to the outside via the rectum.

Colposcopy
Examination of the vagina via a small telescope (colposcope) used in, for example, the removal of cells on the cervix.

Combined Factor
Sub/infertility due to a disorder in both partners.

Conception
The fertilisation of an egg by a single sperm.

Congenital
A condition which is present from birth.

Contraception
The prevention of conception with drugs, barrier methods, intra-uterine devices (IUDs) or 'natural' methods (herbs, timed intercourse, etc.).

Corpus Luteum
The 'yellow body' secreting progesterone which develops in the follicle after it has released an egg.

Cryopreservation
The preservation of tissue (in this context sperm and embryos) by freezing in liquid nitrogen.

Cyst
A capsule of fluid, fat or semi-solid matter.

Cystic Fibrosis
A genetically inherited disorder causing severe damage to digestive organs.

Donor
In this context, a person who donates eggs or sperm, or a couple who donate embryos, for the use of others in ART.

Down's Syndrome
A birth defect resulting from an extra chromosome in the pair 21, resulting in mild to severe learning difficulties.

DNA
(Deoxyribonucleic acid); that part of the cell which contains and transmits genetic (hereditary) information.

Ectopic Pregnancy
A pregnancy occurring outside the womb. The fertilised ovum attaches itself most commonly in the Fallopian tube, but may occasionally stray into the abdominal cavity.

Egg
Female sex cell (also 'ovum', 'female gamete' and 'oocyte').

Egg Collection
The 'harvesting' of eggs from the ovaries following superovulation treatment in IVF. The operation can be done with local or general anaesthetic, either with a laparoscope or by means of inserting an aspiration needle through the vaginal wall.

Egg Donation
The process of giving your own eggs for another's use.

Egg Sharing
Two women sharing one woman's supply of eggs in a given cycle of IVF treatment.

Ejaculate
Seminal fluid expelled from the penis during ejaculation.

Embryo
The fertilised egg up until its eighth week of gestation, after which it is known as a foetus.

Embryo Selection
The choice of embryos for use in IVF.

Embryo Transfer (ET)
The operation in IVF where up to three embryos are transferred to the woman's uterus via a catheter inserted vaginally.

Endocrine Glands
Hormone-secreting glands, including the adrenals, pancreas and – vital to reproduction – the pituitary, ovaries, testicles (and parathyroids).

Endocrine System
The system by which the hormones secreted by the endocrine glands interact with each other and the rest of the body.

Endocrinologist
A hormone specialist.

Endometrial Biopsy
Removal of a small section of tissue in the womb lining for analysis.

Endometriosis
Female condition where endometrial cells grow abnormally outside the womb, causing internal bleeding, pain and reduced fertility.

Endometrium
Lining of the womb, which alters during the menstrual cycle and sheds during menstruation.

Epididymis
Coiled tubing outside the testicles which store sperm.

Erection
Engorgement of erectile tissue in penis or clitoris with blood; a sign of sexual arousal.

ET
See **Embryo Transfer**

Eugenics
Literally 'well born', the manipulation of human genetics for the purpose of producing fitter babies.

Fallopian Tube
Tube leading from the ovary to the uterus which transports the egg to the uterus.

Female Factor
Sub- or infertility due to a disorder in the woman.

Fertilisation
When a sperm successfully burrows into an egg.

Fertility
Ability to produce children.

Fertility Drugs
Hormones used in fertility treatment derived from or analogous to hormones found in the endocrine system.

Fibroid
Benign tumour which can be found in the uterus. It may or may not lead to pregnancy complications.

Fimbria
Finger-like projections at the end of the Fallopian tube which collect the egg after it has been released from the ovary.

Foetus
A developing baby in the womb over eight weeks old.

Follicle
The small sac in the ovary which contains the egg.

Follicle Stimulating Hormone (FSH)
A hormone released by the pituitary gland which in women causes the egg to ripen and in men is essential for healthy sperm development.

Gamete
A sperm or egg.

Gamete Intrafallopian Transfer (GIFT)
The treatment whereby eggs and sperm are mixed outside the body and immediately transferred to the woman's Fallopian tube for normal fertilisation to take place.

Gene
A unit of heredity found on a chromosome.

Genetic Screening
In this context, the screening out of embryos for genetic disorder prior to implantation.

Genito-urinary Tract
The reproductive and excretory systems.

GIFT
See **Gamete Intrafallopian Transfer**

Gonadotrophins
Reproductive hormones from the pituitary gland.

Gonads
Ovaries and testicles.

Gonorrhoea
A bacterial infection and sexually transmitted disease (VD).

Gynaecologist
A specialist in the female reproductive system.

Haemorrhage
Uncontrolled bleeding.

Hormone
Chemical messenger secreted by the endocrine glands. Also made synthetically to mimic natural hormones.

Hormone Replacement Therapy (HRT)
Supplementation of oestrogen for post-menopausal women.

Hostile Mucus
See **Mucus Hostility**

Hot Flushes
Sudden rise in body temperature (as in the menopause) which can also be a side-effect of the drug Buserelin which inhibits pituitary function.

Human Chorionic Gonadotrophins (hCG)
A hormone secreted by the placenta in pregnancy, the presence of which in blood tests confirms pregnancy. Also used in infertility treatment in conjunction with other hormones. Known as the 'midnight injection' in IVF treatment, prior to egg collection.

Human Fertilisation and Embryology Authority (HFEA)
Government quango set up following the passing of the Human
Fertilisation and Embryology Act 1990. A committee of 21 members
regulates the practice of ART in the UK. HFEA licensed clinics are those
clinics in the UK which are authorised by the HFEA to carry out certain
specified fertility treatments.

Human Menopausal Gonadotrophin (hMG)
A follicle-stimulating hormone extracted from the urine of post-menopausal
women for use in fertility treatment (brand name Pergonal).

Humegon
Brand name for drug containing FSH for ovarian stimulation.

Hydrosalpinges
Swelling and blockage of the Fallopian tubes.

Hydrosalpinx
Water on the Fallopian tube caused by hydrosalpinges.

Hyperstimulation
Over-stimulation of ovaries following superovulation drug treatment.

Hypothalamus
The part of the brain which controls the pituitary, which releases LH and
FSH hormones in men and women.

Hysterosalpingogram (HSG)
X-ray study of the uterus and Fallopian tubes using a dye injected into the
uterus.

Hysteroscopy
Inspection of the womb cavity using a hysteroscope.

ICSI
See **Intra-cytoplasmic Sperm Injection**

Immotile
Not moving (used in reference to sperm which don't swim).

Implantation
The attachment of the embryo to the uterine wall.

Impotence
A man's inability to produce or sustain erection.

Incision
A surgical cut.

Infertility Counselling
Specialist counselling on the medical, ethical and emotional implications of infertility treatment.

Intracytoplasmic Sperm Injection (ICSI)
Very recent technique of injecting a single sperm into the egg for *in vitro* fertilisation (IVF).

Intrauterine
Within the uterus.

Intrauterine Device (IUD)
A contraceptive device inserted in the uterus.

Intrauterine Insemination (IUI)
Fresh (that is, unfrozen) sperm (from partner or donor) is washed and introduced into the womb via a catheter.

In Vitro Fertilisation (IVF)
Fertilisation of the egg by the sperm outside the body in laboratory conditions (prior to being replaced in the womb).

In Vitro Maturation (IVM)
The collection of immature egg(s) and developing it/them *in vitro* to maturity for fertilisation.

Involuntary Childlessness
A desire for children that is inhibited by sub- or infertility.

Isthmus
Part of Fallopian tube closest to uterus.

IVF Unit
(HFEA-licensed) clinic specialising in IVF techniques.

Klinefelter's Syndrome
Condition where the man has an extra X chromosome, usually resulting in sterility (absence of sperm in semen).

Labia Majora
Large lips of the vagina which cover the vagina and surrounding area.

Labia Minora
Small lips of the vagina which are part of the vulva and cover the vaginal opening.

Lactation
The production of milk in the breast, governed by endocrine hormones.

Laparoscopy
Examination of the pelvic organs with a laparoscope (telescope) inserted surgically through the abdomen. (The procedure is also known as 'Lap and Dye' because of the dye used to test tubal patency.)

Laparotomy
Tubal surgery.

League Tables
Published success rates of treatments by clinics.

Liquid Nitrogen
Chemical used to freeze sperm and embryos.

Luteal Phase
The second phase of the menstrual cycle after ovulation when the corpus luteum is producing progesterone.

Luteinising Hormone (LH)
Hormone secreted in the pituitary gland. In women it is produced during the menstrual cycle to stimulate the production of progesterone in the corpus luteum. In men it stimulates the production of testosterone in the testicles.

Male Factor
Sub- or infertility due to a disorder in the man.

Menarche
First menstrual period.

Menstrual Cycle
Woman's reproductive cycle occurring over approximately 28 days during which the ovary releases an egg and the womb lining prepares to receive the egg (if fertilised) or to shed it (if not).

Menstruation
Bleeding at the end of a menstrual cycle.

MESA
See **Microsurgical Epididymal Sperm Aspiration**

Metrodin High Purity
Brand name for the follicle-stimulating hormone hMG.

Microinjection
Injection of single sperm into egg (*see* **ICSI**).

Microinsemination (MIST)
See **ICSI**

Microsurgery
Surgery performed with the use of microscopes on minute parts of the human body, such as the Fallopian tubes.

Microsurgical Epididymal Sperm Aspiration (MESA)
Procedure whereby sperm is aspirated directly from the epididymis to be used in IVF/ICSI in cases where the man has vasal blockage or absence.

Mid-cycle
Point in the woman's menstrual cycle when ovulation should occur.

Miscarriage
Spontaneous loss of pregnancy.

Motility
In this context, sperm's ability to move.

Mucus Hostility
Condition where the woman's cervical mucus is actually killing off her partner's sperm before it gets a chance to swim up the cervical canal to reach the egg.

Multiple Pregnancy
A pregnancy of one or more foetuses.

Normospermia
Normal semen analysis.

Obstetrician
Specialist in pregnancy care.

Oestrogen
Female sex hormone secreted in ovaries, but also in the adrenals of both men and women.

Oligozoospermia (Oligospermia)
Poor sperm count (such as less than 20 million per ml).

Oocyte
Immature egg.

Orgasm
Climax of pleasure in sexual intercourse. In men produces ejaculation of semen; in women, vaginal and uterine contractions.

Ovarian Hyperstimulation Syndrome (OHSS)
Serious but rare condition where, following superovulation drug treatment, there is a build-up of fluid in the abdomen, thorax and sometimes the sac surrounding the heart, and thrombosis in the veins and arteries. Heart attack, stroke or loss of limb can result.

Ovarian Stimulation/Induction
The stimulation of the ovaries to produce eggs, either when the ovaries are underactive or – in ART – to cause superovulation artificially.

Ovarian Tissue
Tissue from the ovary which can be used to nurture eggs to full development for use in IVF.

Ovulation
The release of the egg from the ovary triggered by a surge in the luteinising hormone.

Ovum
Mature egg (plural ova).

Patency
In this context, openness (as in Fallopian tubal patency).

Patient Support Group
A support group attached to a fertility clinic.

Pelvic Inflammatory Disease (PID)
Infection of the reproductive organs in a woman. Can lead to scarring and adhesions in tubes, contributing to subfertility. Most common cause of female factor infertility.

Percutaneous Epididymal Sperm Aspiration (PESA)
Retrieving sperm directly from the epididymis using a needle.

Pergonal
Brand name for drug containing 50% FSH and 50% LH to stimulate the ovary to produce eggs. Used in IVF treatment.

PESA
See **Percutaneous Epididymal Sperm Aspiration**

Pituitary Gland
Gland located at the base of the brain which is responsible for major hormone secretions including FSH and LH, which are key players in the reproductive hormone system.

Polycystic Ovaries
Presence of cysts in the ovaries which may not necessarily affect fertility.

Polycystic Ovary Syndrome (PCOS)
Condition in which ovarian cysts do inhibit fertility.

Post-Coital Test
A test performed on the sperm and cervical mucus after intercourse to check for mucus hostility and sperm survival.

Pre-embryo
An embryo up until 14 days, or when the 'primitive streak' occurs.

Pregnancy
The successful implantation of the embryo in the uterus and subsequent gestation of the baby *in utero* until birth. (*NB:* In IVF, a 'pregnancy result' might be the result of early testing and can refer to an implantation when hormone levels are insufficient to ensure the continuation of the pregnancy. Miscarriage would certainly follow.)

Pre-implantation
First five days or so of an embryo's development prior to implantation in the womb lining.

Pre-implantation Genetic Diagnosis
The analysis of pre-embryos to screen out inherited genetic disorders.

Premature Ejaculation
Ejaculation of semen too early in sexual intercourse, resulting in loss of erection.

Premature Menopause
Condition where a woman ceases to ovulate and has her menopause before it its due. This can start at 30 years old or earlier.

Primary Infertility
Never having had a pregnancy.

Primitive Streak
The first sign in the embryo of the development of a nervous system.

Progesterone
Female reproductive hormone secreted by the corpus luteum and other organs during pregnancy.

Prolactin
Hormone secreted in the pituitary which stimulates the milk-producing glands.

Prostate Gland
The male gland which contributes a major portion of the fluid which makes up semen.

Reproductive Technology
Medical and surgical techniques for achieving reproduction without sex (the opposite of contraception).

Reprogenetics
The combination of reproductive medicine and genetics.

Retroversion of the Uterus
Condition where the uterus is angled backwards.

Salpingitis
Inflammation of the Fallopian tubes following infection.

Salpingogram
X-ray of the Fallopian tubes.

Salpingoplasty
Surgical repair of the Fallopian tubes.

Salpingostomy
Surgical operation to open the Fallopian tubes near the fimbria (that is, at ovary end).

Secondary Infertility
Cases of infertility where a pregnancy has previously occurred and a child(ren) has/have been born.

Semen
Fluid of the male ejaculate including sperm and other secretions.

Semen Analysis
Test for sperm motility, morphology and density.

Seminal Vesicles
Glands which produce an acidic fluid making up more than half of the semen in a male ejaculate.

Seminiferous
Seed-carrying.

Seminiferous Tubules
Long tubes in the testes in which the sperm are formed.

Serono
One of the largest drug manufacturers specialising in infertility drugs.

Sex Selection
The screening out of embryos of a certain gender for medical or social reasons.

Spermatid
Immature sperm. Also refers to technique where an immature sperm is injected into the egg (currently illegal in the UK).

Spermatozoon (sperm)
Fully developed male reproductive cell.

Sperm Bank
Clinic where donors give sperm and where it is stored.

Sperm Count
See **Semen Analysis**

Spermicide
A substance which kills sperm, for example as is added to condoms.

Sperm Preparation
The preparation of sperm for treatment in Assisted Conception.

Spinnbarkeit
Stringy stretchability of cervical mucus.

Spontaneous Abortion
Miscarriage.

Spontaneous Pregnancy
A pregnancy achieved without ART.

Standardised Selective Salpingography (SSS)
Use of hysterosalpingogram and catheterisation to clear out debris in the Fallopian tubes. A substitute for surgery.

Sterile
Permanently infertile.

Sterilisation
Procedure to halt fertility.

Subfertility
A problem, not necessarily untreatable, which inhibits conception.

Sub-zonal Insemination (SUZI)
Method similar to ICSI in which a single sperm is injected into the zona, next to the egg.

Surrogacy
The use of a third party (woman) to gestate a baby and give birth to it for a woman who has no womb. Can involve use of the surrogate's womb only, with an embryo implantation, or can involve the use of her eggs, inseminated by the male of the recipient couple.

SUZI
See **Sub-zonal Insemination**

Swim-up Test
Test to check sperm's motility after it has been washed in a laboratory.

'Take-home Baby'
A live baby born from ART.

Temperature Chart
Chart to monitor the woman's body temperature in order to ascertain ovulation.

TESE
See **Testicular Sperm Extraction**

Testes
Testicles or male gonads.

Testicular Sperm Extraction (TESE)
Sperm removed directly from the testis.

Testosterone
Male sex hormone secreted in the testes.

'Test-tube' Baby
Popular term for a baby fertilised *in vitro*.

Tubal Insufflation
Test for tubal patency involving the blowing of gas through the Fallopian tubes.

Turner's Syndrome
A female condition in which a sex chromosome is absent, causing infertility.

Ultrasound (Ultrasound Scan)
A diagnostic device that uses sound waves rather than x-rays to visualise the body. Can be done on the abdomen or vaginally.

Unexplained Infertility
Cases where no pathology is found in either partner yet pregnancy isn't occurring.

Urethra
Tube which takes urine out of the body.

Uterine
Relating to the uterus.

Uterine Cavity/Uterus
The womb.

Vagina
Birth canal.

Vaginismus
Condition where the muscles around the vaginal opening contract in spasms making intercourse painful or impossible.

Varicole
Varicose condition of the scrotal veins, which may cause infertility (can be treated surgically).

Vas Deferens
The tube which links the epididymis to the prostate gland.

Vasectomy
Surgical tying of the vas deferens to produce voluntary sterilisation.

Venereal Disease
Sexually transmitted disease/infection.

Vulva
Area outside the vagina.

ZIFT
See **Zygote Intrafallopian Transfer**

Zona pellucida
The shell of the human egg.

Zygote
A fertilised egg.

Zygote Intrafallopian Transfer (ZIFT)
Similar to GIFT, except here it is fertilised embryos which are transferred to the Fallopian tubes while the woman is under general anaesthetic.

References

Introduction

I. Office of Population Census and Surveys 1991, quoted in *Family Policy Studies Centre News Release*, 10th April, 1995.

Chapter 2: State of the ART

I. Carl Djerassi, *Menachem's Same* (Zurich: Haffmans Verlag, 1996). Novelist Carl Djerassi is the chemist who invented the contraceptive pill. This excerpt reveals the voice of one of his central characters, Melanie Laidlaw, director of REPCON, a foundation for research into reproductive medicine. Melanie, single, 'mature' and childless, eventually 'steals' her (married) infertile lover's sperm and has his baby by ICSI.
At the time of writing, this novel is not yet published in English.
II. *British Medical Journal* 299 (1988): pages 309–11.
III. Multiple Births Foundation Annual Report, 1995.
IV. HFEA 5th Annual Report, 1996.
V. Each Consultant in charge and his/her team will have their own views and 'style' of treatment reflected in the drug combinations and doses, as well as a policy of 'tailoring' prescriptions to suit the individual.
VI. Sammy Lee, *Counselling in Male Infertility* (Blackwell Science, 1996).

Chapter 3: Feelings

I. HF & E Act 1990 s 13(6); schedule 3 para 3(1) (a).
II. HFEA Code of Practice 1995. Part 6 (6.4.): pages 31–2.

Chapter 4: Access

I. Report of the Third National Survey of NHS Funding of Infertility Services, July 95. National Infertility Awareness Campaign.
II. Professor Robert Winston, *Making Babies* (BBC Books, 1996).
III. *The Observer*, 4th June 1995.
IV. Ibid.
V. Ibid.

Chapter 6: Adoption and Fostering

I. Marriage and Divorce Statistics Series. FM2, OPCS 1992.
II. This digest of PAL principles was quoted in *MOSAIC* (Summer 1995).
III. Adoption – A service for Children. Adoption Bill – A consultative document. Department of Health Welsh Office, March 1996.

Chapter 7: The Body Politic

I. HFEA 5th Annual Report, 1996.
II. *The Observer*, 4th June 1995.
III. Abortion Act 1967 Chapter 87 1 – (1) (b).
IV. *Ivy's Genes*, an Isis film for Channel 4, directed by Sarah Boston.
V. Sammy Lee, *Counselling in Male Infertility* (Blackwell Science, 1996.
VI. The Board for Social Responsibility, *Personal Origins* (2nd edn; CHP, 1996).
VII. HFEA Code of Practice Part 3 3.14: page 13.
VIII. +, July 1996.

Index